FERTILITY COOKBOOK

Author
Associate Prof. Hakan COKSUER

Translated by
Gonul Uguralp Cannon

Editorial Consultant
Mursel Cavus

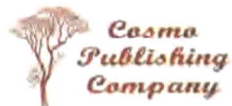

Publisher

Cosmo Publishing Company

ISBN: 978-1-949872-07-1

All rights reserved, including the rights of reproduction in whole or in part of any form

THE RELATIONSHIP BETWEEN NUTRITION AND FERTILITY	I
Preparation for Pregnancy	II
Psychological and Mental Preparation for the Diet	IV
How Proper Nutrition Can Increase Your Fertility	V
Proper Nutrition: The Initial Condition for Healthy Reproduction	VIII
DETAILS ON COOKING TECHNIQUES	X
Boiling	X
Cooking slowly by poaching	X
Sautéing	XI
Baking	XI
Braising	XI
Steaming	XI
Suggestions on Cooking Legumes	XII
BUYING THE COOKWARE	XIII
SELECTING HEALTHY FOOD	XIV
What should we pay attention to when choosing our food?	XV
HOW TO CHOOSE AND PRESERVE VEGETABLES	XVI
CHOOSING FRUITS	XIX
WHAT KIND OF CONTAINERS KEEP FOOD "FRESH AND NUTRITIOUS"?	XX
HOW TO CUT AND SLICE FOOD	XXI
Should I use a knife to cut greens?	XXI
Should bamboo, plastic or ceramic knives be preferred?	XXII
Should we use a blender?	XXII
THINGS TO KNOW ABOUT VEGETABLES	XXII
How should fresh vegetables be cooked?	XXII
Make your salad healthy and tasty	XXIII
Washing vegetables	XXIII
Preparing the vegetables	XXIV
Storage life of vegetables	XXIV
Cutting the vegetables	XXIV
Extending the life of vegetables	XXV
Prepare delicious vegetable dishes with their vibrant colors!	XXV
Practical hints	XXVI
HYGIENE IN THE KITCHEN	XXVI
Do not forget these	XXVIII
THINGS YOU NEED TO CONSIDER IN YOUR NUTRITION	XXVIII

RECIPES

ASSOCIATE PROF. HAKAN COKSUER 1
THE RELATIONSHIP BETWEEN NUTRITION AND FERTILITY I

Preparation for Pregnancy II

Psychological and Mental Preparation for the Diet IV

How Proper Nutrition Can Increase Your Fertility V

Proper Nutrition: The Initial Condition for Healthy Reproduction VIII
DETAILS ON COOKING TECHNIQUES X

Boiling X

Cooking slowly by poaching X

Sautéing XI

Baking XI

Braising XI

Steaming XI

Suggestions on Cooking Legumes XII
BUYING THE COOKWARE XIII
SELECTING HEALTHY FOOD XIV

What should we pay attention to when choosing our food? XV
HOW TO CHOOSE AND PRESERVE VEGETABLES XVI
CHOOSING FRUITS XIX
WHAT KIND OF CONTAINERS KEEP FOOD "FRESH AND NUTRITIOUS"? XX
HOW TO CUT AND SLICE FOOD XXI

Should I use a knife to cut greens? XXI

Should bamboo, plastic or ceramic knives be preferred? XXII

Should we use a blender? XXII
THINGS TO KNOW ABOUT VEGETABLES... XXII

How should fresh vegetables be cooked? XXII

Make your salad healthy and tasty XXIII

Washing vegetables XXIII

Preparing the vegetables XXIV

Storage life of vegetables XXIV

Cutting the vegetables XXIV

Extending the life of vegetables XXV

Prepare delicious vegetable dishes with their vibrant colors! XXV

Practical hints XXVI

- To prevent apples from spoiling in the fridge, do not let them touch one another and keep the stem parts upright. XXVI

- Wet your knife in hot water to prevent your hard-boiled egg from smearing. Do not dry your knife before slicing the egg. XXVI

- You can use the same method for slicing fresh bread, but this time dry the knife immediately after soaking it in hot water. With this method, you will be able to cut the bread without wrecking the loaf. XXVI

- You should toss dried fruits and nuts in flour to prevent them from sinking to the bottom when you make a cake with those ingredients. You will see that coating with flour helps them distribute evenly throughout the batter. XXVI

- Put a cup of water under the grill to avoid smoke when you have a barbecue at home. Water absorbs both the smoke and the oil. XXVI

HYGIENE IN THE KITCHEN XXVI

Do not forget these XXVIII

- There's no need to avoid oils or fats. We should consume oils or fats as naturally as possible, as we consume other foods. XXVIII

- Oils are sensitive to heat. You should consume oils in their natural state without allowing any formation of trans fats. XXVIII

- Our body does not produce Omega 3 or Omega 6 fats. We need to get them from foods that are rich in them, as both help to maintain a comfortable pregnancy as well as to promote the neurodevelopment of the baby. XXVIII

- Olive oil is of great value, but be careful to use oil without over-heating it. Choose an olive oil produced by traditional methods. .. XXVIII
THINGS YOU NEED TO CONSIDER IN YOUR NUTRITION XXVIII

THE RELATIONSHIP BETWEEN NUTRITION AND FERTILITY

For fertility, the way couples eat is as important as the medical treatment. Women who eat healthfully can produce healthy eggs as they maintain their insulin hormone level within normal range. It's important also to remember the advantages of exercise in keeping insulin at its normal level. As you use the recipes in this book, you should also pay attention to exercise. If you are trying to get pregnant, you should work on improving your diet at least three months in advance.

To regulate fertility functions, the kind of carbohydrates you're consuming is an important factor. Consumption of grains, legumes, and fruits, which are sources of good nutrition, increases the possibility of conception; consumption of carbohydrates like white sugar and fruit juice decreases fertility functions.

The best protein sources to boost fertility include eggs, fatty fish, grains, nuts, and seeds. The consumption of such proteins can promote fertility.

For fertility, the body needs fats to a certain extent, and it is not correct to identify all kinds of fats as harmful. Fatty acids that are found in nuts, seeds, and fatty fish are necessary for fertility. Omega-3 fats, which are found in fatty fish, especially in salmon, mackerel, and sardines, are essential not only for fertility but also for general health. The consumption of pre-packaged meals that include trans fatty acids should be restricted, because those trans fats affect fertility in a negative way. Staying away from processed food like salami and sausage, canned food, organ meats, deli products, fried food, sugar and all kinds of pastry is a general rule that we usually hear. Are you ready to hear even more?

Preparation for Pregnancy

You may be asking yourself: Why do I need a cookbook to facilitate pregnancy? Cleansing a woman's body of toxins during the pre-conception period increases the chances of conception and healthy growth of the baby from the very first moment. Although future mothers think that developing "a pregnancy dietary habit" is similar to eating properly for their own health, it is not exactly the same.

A pregnancy diet is designed to promote the health of both the mother and the baby, as well as maximize the fertility of the mother. These recipes and the nutrition style outlined in this book represent a diet for all women who are preparing themselves for the miracle of pregnancy, whether they have a fertility issue or not. To achieve maximum results, future mothers should use these recipes as well as apply some basic lifestyle principles. Therefore, you can consider this book a sequel to **Pregnancy Diet for Perfect Babies.** However, if you did not read that book, I would like to say a little about that diet.

There are several important key points about this diet. First, it includes different nutrition groups, such as proteins, carbohydrates, and fats, in a balanced way. Second, it consists of slow-digesting foods. And third, it supports general health and increases fertility. In order to align with all these key points, we also paid attention to the recipes we created so that they are easy to cook, doable with ingredients on hand, and rich in variety. On top of that, we wanted to include in our book all the details you need to carefully consider while preparing your food, thinking holistically.

One of the most important characteristics of this diet is that it keeps blood sugar stable after and in between meals. Our goal, with the help of slow-digesting foods, is to inhibit the rapid conversion of food into sugar by insulin and glucagon hormones, regulate blood sugar, and decrease the risk of insulin resistance. This helps to eliminate problems arising from hormones and ovary issues. In other words, what is essential is not to avoid the consumption of sugar or carbohydrates but to avoid the fluctuation of blood sugar levels during the day, to maintain hormonal balance.

You can consider this style of nutrition as your new lifestyle. You should first go over your cooking habits one by one and gain new habits. Before starting the diet, get all the pre-packaged food out of your kitchen and out of your life, because once you start your diet, you need to stay away from everything that would either tempt you to revert to old habits or distract you. Once you clear your kitchen of those foods you will no longer consume, replace them with our suggestions! You will realize that you will feel much more energetic and contented as you enjoy these recipes and foods.

Try to consume fruits and vegetables seasonally. Nuts are healthy snacks as long as they are not eaten in large portions. Making your own yogurt at home will not only give you joy but also enable you to include a healthy food in your meal. Plus, it is so easy! Of course, it is important that the milk you make yogurt with is from a good dairy farm, and fresh. Do not forget, each detail is essential, and those details altogether add up in our daily lives. Don't say, "Who cares if I don't make my yogurt at home?" because that is not a helpful approach. You have made a decision to change your life. You are now a different person and soon will become a mother.

Psychological and Mental Preparation for the Diet

Fertility Cookbook for Perfect Babies will guide you during your preparation period for pregnancy, which is an exciting process. You will have a healthier body and baby with the help of this book. The information I will share is based on things that every person should practice having a healthy life. Besides, since the intention is not to change your body weight, my suggestions will not be challenging. I only ask you to change your habits one by one. I also do not force you to consume any food that you do not want or are not used to. On the contrary, I just advise simple changes so that you can give birth to a healthy baby. Considering the nutrition style of the Turkish culture, my team and I selected the foods that you can find in the produce section or at a farmer's market so that you can easily follow the diet. We planned everything with the thought that a diet list is not easy to get, and without a list, it is difficult to follow the diet. Okay, then, how can you put our suggestions into practice?

1. At the end of the book, you will make *a list of things that you need to change.* As you read our suggestions, write down everything that does not suit your lifestyle or habits, and in the same space also note what you need to change, as well as how you will change it. For example, if you use two cutting boards, note that you need to buy a third one.

2. Put a note on the refrigerator or at another attention-grabbing spot in the kitchen for the suggestions you think are necessary to include in your daily life and that you might forget. In fact, put a reminder on your phone.

3. Developing a lifelong habit is not an easy process; some days, in the midst of intensive work, you may skip or ignore it. Don't be upset with yourself at that stage, and say, "I promise myself that I will be more determined from now on." You don't need to be angry at yourself, but you do need to change yourself.

How Proper Nutrition Can Increase Your Fertility

It is claimed that what's needed for human life to begin is **two cells and a miracle.** A critical balance of hormones and physiological changes in a female body cause that miracle to occur. Of course, the influence of men, as much as women, in this miracle is indisputable.

During the preconception and prenatal period, the female body goes through a fairly critical and complicated process. This process causes complex hormonal changes: some parts of the brain secrete hormones, some are carried in the blood, organs produce hormones, and then there are the effects of other organs responding to these changes. All of these complex changes support and trigger one another. Fertility, in its basic and most common definition, is the ability of a woman to get pregnant, and the ability of a man to impregnate a woman. The first stage of pregnancy before the fertilization of two cells is the release of a mature egg by the ovaries to the fallopian tube and the regulation of this process by a balanced hormone system. In other words, we can say that hormones and their carriers are the key performers that influence a successful ovulation and sperm production. Still, you may be questioning the connection between fertility and nutrition!

Let's look at those hormones and carriers that are important to us in order to better understand the effects of nutrition on fertility. We can think of hormones as team players who not only score a goal for fertility but also help us make perfect babies. For example, FSH and LH hormones take major roles in regulating fertility. Estrogen, on the other hand, causes the growth and thickening of the endometrium tissue, which lines the inner cavity of the uterus and enables implantation of the fertilized egg to the uterine lining. It also gets the uterus ready and prepares a safe home for the egg, which keeps dividing into cells as it floats down the fallopian tube to the uterus, where it can implant and develop. *Progesterone*, which affects the ovulation pattern, supports estrogen in stimulating endometrium tissue to grow.

Insulin is a hormone produced by the pancreas and plays an essential role in regulating blood sugar. It is also important for fertility. Instant rises in the blood sugar level alert the pancreas and cause the secretion of insulin. A high level of insulin inhibits the function of globulin, and as a result, globulin cannot sufficiently control testosterone, a male hormone present in the blood. A high level of testosterone hormone circulating freely leads to undesirable effects on female reproductive health; it prevents having babies!

Is that all? Of course not. High levels of insulin and testosterone also affect our health, and at the same time can cause ovarian cysts, also called polycystic ovary syndrome (PCOS), which prevents ovulation. One other hormone that affects fertility is *leptin, a* hormone released from fat cells. After storing fat and getting swollen, that is, having eaten enough food, fat cells secrete leptin and send signals signaling saturation. Studies show that long-term fasting and decrease in leptin levels have effects on the reproductive system. Fasting for a long period may reduce ovulation in women and sperm production in men. You can prepare your body for the miracle of pregnancy and eliminate these negative effects by eating regularly and avoiding long-term fasting.

Proper Nutrition: The Initial Condition for Healthy Reproduction

The level of hormones we referred to previously and the way they work can be strongly affected by our nutritional habits. Nutrition is a complicated process! Why? Because, starting from the minute you take a bite in your mouth, the process, which includes the interaction of the food with enzymes in the saliva and digestive processes in the stomach and the intestines, is affected by many factors. It is surprising to see that the amount and variety of sugar contained in the foods we consume, although no harm or toxic effects are mentioned in the labeling, can affect ovulation. Many factors, such as cooking styles, beverages, side dishes, and portion sizes contribute to how our bodies use these foods.

Besides making changes such as avoiding regular heavy exercise, smoking, alcohol, foods containing added hormones, and pre-packaged and ready-made foods, it is important that you follow your diet and "eat healthy" not only to prepare your body for a healthy pregnancy but also to hold a healthy baby in your arms at the end of about 40 weeks. As a physician, I advise you to take the time to think about and change your eating habits.

Actually, nature programmed the female body to perform a miracle and bring life to the world. What you need to do is to take good care of your body and pay attention to a healthy diet.

We have created the recipes in this book to increase your fertility. I recommend starting your diet three months before you hope to get pregnant. It is important to take the vitamins and other supplements that your doctor prescribes during your regular visits for the continuity of your pregnancy and the health of your baby.

You should make sure that all the food you buy for your diet does not affect your health negatively. Our priority is heirloom seeds and organic nutrients! Another important aspect is to cook fruits and vegetables, after washing them carefully, in a way that they do not lose their nutrition and vitamin value. How you store foods, whether cooked or uncooked, to preserve their nutritive value is also important.

For this reason, beyond what's generally included in a simple "recipe book," we have provided information that will prepare you to become healthier and more fertile individuals.

Eat well and healthy and have a perfect baby!

DETAILS ON COOKING TECHNIQUES

Before diving into cooking techniques, let's remember the most important ways to remove toxins occurring in foods. Not all toxins remain active during cooking. Some toxins, like botulism, become inactivated by cooking. Boiling food for 10 minutes kills this toxin. Nonetheless, many toxins are resistant to heat. To prevent toxins from being produced, do not keep food at room temperature for more than two hours. On hot days, food should not be left out for more than an hour. Cooking techniques are crucial to avoid generating trans fats as a result of overheated oil, to retain the nutritional value of foods and to have a healthier kitchen.

Boiling

Boiling is often used in cooking meats, vegetables, grains, and legumes. Because it is one of the healthiest cooking techniques, it is very much preferred. Since nutrients of boiled foods leach into the water, the cooking water tastes good, and I advise you to drink it. You can also prepare soups and sauces by adding various spices to the boiling water.

Cooking slowly by poaching

Poaching is a technique of cooking food in dry or wet steam, either with pressure or without pressure. It's an excellent technique for cooking fish. Since it involves no oil, cooking is healthier with this technique. Compared to boiling, you're less likely to lose vitamins and minerals from leaching into water.

Sautéing

Sautéing is used to cook small and finely cut pieces of food quickly. Cooking with the sautéing technique, which requires constant stirring, prevents food from giving out natural juices, and thus the nutritional elements of the food are preserved.

Baking

This is one of the easiest techniques of cooking. Once the prepared food is placed in a baking pan and the oven is set to the desired temperature, the cooking process begins. The important point here is not to overcook the food. Since the food will be cooked with the fat and water it contains, there is no need for extra water or oil.

Braising

Using a tightly covered vessel, you can cook the food either in the oven or in a pan on the stovetop with little water.

Steaming

The smell, taste, color and texture of any meat, fish, fruits, or vegetables in a dish is better preserved by steaming than boiling. Cooking with steam is one of the top techniques that minimize the loss of nutritional elements.

- It is the best cooking technique for fish and vegetables.
- When cooked with steam, the starch in the food softens and causes the vegetable to become tender.
- It promotes digestion.
- The color, texture, appearance, and smell of food does not change.

- It preserves the unique flavor and appearance of vegetables.
- It minimizes the loss of soluble nutritional elements, retains nutritional value (it's the technique that results in the least loss of vitamins and minerals), and reduces protein denaturation to a minimum.

Suggestions on Cooking Legumes

You will remember how often I included legumes in the sample recipes in our book, **Pregnancy *Diet for Perfect Babies*.** Dried legumes, which are rich in vitamins and minerals, are among the most important fiber sources. However, if not cooked carefully, they can lose a lot of their vitamin, mineral and nutritional value. You should keep the following in mind while cooking legumes.

- Store legumes away from windows, sunlight, and cooking areas.
- To check the freshness of your legumes, put a few in some water. Fresh legumes sink, old ones float.
- If you are pre-boiling the legume before cooking, do not add salt to the boiling water.
- Adding a pinch of sodium bicarbonate to the boiling water will speed cooking.
- Legumes should be soaked in water at least eight hours before cooking. It is necessary to pour off this liquid, since components that cause intestinal gas leach into the water. However, do not pour off the cooking water, to avoid vitamin and mineral loss.
- If you forget to soak your legumes ahead of time, boil them for five minutes and then allow them to cool for

an hour with the lid on the pan. The effect is the same as soaking.

• If you are cooking the legumes to be used for a salad, let them sit in the water they were boiled in to cool. This prevents the skin from coming off and gives the legumes a fresher appearance.

BUYING THE COOKWARE

Since our aim is to get the most nutrition possible out of our foods, we should also take great care without choice of cookware.

Stainless-steel pots and pans: As you choose your pots and pans, make sure the steel is not thin. Cooking in a high-quality stainless-steel cookware is quicker. Foods not only lose less nutritional value but also look and taste better.

Pressure-cooker: Allowing cooking in steam in a shorter period of time, pressure-cookers save time. You can cook dried foods, like legumes, easily with a pressure-cooker.

Glass cookware: Heat-resistant glass pots and pans are among the healthiest types of cookware. Despite the disadvantage of not evenly distributing heat, they are preferable since they do not produce a reaction with nutrients in your food. Using shallow glass cookware will allow for more even cooking. Also, keeping cooked food in glass containers is much healthier.

SELECTING HEALTHY FOOD

We used to eat mainly natural foods until 40 to 50 years ago, but today we have foods on our plates that are genetically modified, rich in chemicals, frozen, and full of harmful substances, and we are mostly unaware of it. Removing toxins by expelling such foods from your kitchen and gravitating to a healthy diet is a cornerstone for the development of your body and your future baby.

So, how do we differentiate healthy foods from unhealthy ones? Although more crops are harvested as a result of industrialization in agriculture, the use of pesticides and chemical fertilizers causes the crops to grow differently.

The production process in which each stage of production is controlled without the use of chemicals, chemical fertilizers, hormones or antibiotics is called **organic agriculture**. A logo is displayed on the products to show that they are produced by organic agriculture. By looking for these logos, you can buy your products from reliable brands.

The World Trade Organization (WTO) has developed agreements on Animal and Plant Health based on food security in international standards. The first agreement on the Application of Sanitary and Phytosanitary Standards (SPS Agreement) is "Hazard Analysis and Critical Control Points" (HACCP) for food, and the other is GAP, which stands for "Good Agricultural Practice," for agricultural production. If the product you buy is not organic, you should at least check whether it is produced with "Good Agricultural Practice" or not.

Also, by producing your own food or buying organic food from trustworthy producers, you can support healthy food production.

What should we pay attention to when choosing our food?

- First of all, eat seasonally.
- The flavor, smell, and nutritional value of seasonal tomatoes are much better than for greenhouse tomatoes. This applies to all vegetables and fruits.
- Like vegetables, fish needs to be eaten in its season. We should stay away from farmed fish as much as possible and try to consume wild-caught ocean fish instead. Compared to farmed fish, ocean fish have higher nutritional value and better quality. Cold-water fish are preferred.
- There is an important detail you need to know about the shelf life of products when you shop at a market. Long or short shelf life, as labeled, does not necessarily show that the product is either good or bad. In order to make sure that the product is produced in an ideal way and arrives to consumers in ideal condition, based on the product features, the producers determine a different shelf life for each product.
- In addition, it is best to choose vacuum-packed products when buying pre-packaged ones, because microorganisms grow in oxygen. Vacuum-packing removes the oxygen. In modified-atmosphere packages,

either nitrogen gas or a nitrogen gas mixture is used. There is no risk of microorganism growth in products packaged in this way.

• You should stay away from food products with color additives. The colorants that we often hear about are quinoline yellow and caramel color. While caramel color is used to give a brownish color, quinoline color is preferred in food products such as snacks, margarine, and cheese.

HOW TO CHOOSE AND PRESERVE VEGETABLES

There is no need to belabor vegetable selection. Knowing a few basic details will help you buy and consume vegetables at the peak of their freshness.

Zucchini: Those firm and dark in color are ideal. Zucchini stays fresh in the refrigerator up to five days.

Broccoli: The freshest broccoli has firm and dense flowers and is dark green. You can keep broccoli fresh in the refrigerator for a week.

Spinach: Spinach with crisp and dark green leaves is fresh. Wrap spinach with a paper towel before storing in the refrigerator. Storing green leafy vegetables in the refrigerator for a long time is not good, so keep spinach in the crisper up to three to four days at the most, and then cook it.

Cucumber: Firm, juicy and bright cucumbers are the freshest. Some of the heirloom types have a spiky skin, which is more natural. You can keep your cucumbers in the crisper drawers of your refrigerator up to five days.

Asparagus: When choosing asparagus, prefer firm stalks with unopened leaves. If you store the asparagus vertically in a jar with a lid, it will stay fresh longer. Still, because asparagus is not a long-lasting vegetable, it is best to cook it as soon as possible.

Okra: Choose more tender pods. Okra can be canned, and it can also be kept fresh in the crisper for three days.

Lettuce: Lettuce with crisp, bright green leaves is fresh. Like spinach, you can wash and wrap lettuce in a paper towel to keep in the crisper. This way, you can keep it fresh up to five days.

Leek: Those with white roots and bright green leaves are fresh. The leaves should not be slimy, but crisp. If the leaves are slimy, you can cut off those parts and store the rest in the crisper drawer for a week.

Onion: The most important thing you need to consider when choosing onions is whether they are dry. Onions with dry skin and no moist spots are ideal. If you keep onions in a dry, cool location, away from sunlight, they can stay fresh up to two months. When you cut and use an onion, you can store the remaining portion in a storage bag in the refrigerator for up to four days.

Potato: The most important tip in selecting potatoes is to choose those that are firm, smooth and have no sprouts.

As long as you keep potatoes in a dry, cool location with no sunlight, they stay fresh for a month. Keep them unwashed until it's time to cook them.

Cabbage: Of winter vegetables, cabbage is one of the most vitamin-rich. Be sure to pick a tight and compact head with light green to white leaves on the outside. You can keep cabbage fresh in the crisper drawer up to weeks.

Carrot: Make sure that carrots are firm and not damaged. Carrots stay fresh in the crisper drawer up to two weeks.

Tomato: Firm and ripe tomatoes are the freshest. You can save your tomatoes in the crisper of the refrigerator, but they'll taste better if you keep them in a dry and cool location away from sunlight.

Cauliflower: Make sure cauliflower heads are firm, bright in color and free of blemishes. You can keep cauliflower fresh in the crisper drawer for a week.

Eggplant: If the skin is bright and dark purple, and the stem is bright green, the eggplant is at its peak of freshness. Avoid choosing the softest ones and try not to buy firm ones that might be unripe. You can keep eggplant in the crisper drawer of the refrigerator for up to five days.

Garlic: Pick unblemished and taut-skinned bulbs. You can store them fresh in a cool and dry area away from sunlight for up to two months.

CHOOSING FRUITS

Banana: You can find the freshest bananas in January and February. They'll stay fresh up to five days in the open at room temperature.

Apple: The best time for picking fresh apples from the tree is September and October. Make sure apples you buy are firm, with smooth skin.

Grapes: Grape harvest begins in July and lasts until October. Grapes stay fresh in the crisper drawer for three days.

Oranges: November, December, and January are the orange season months. Oranges can be stored for a week at room temperature and two weeks in the refrigerator.

Strawberry: You can start eating strawberries from the beginning of the season in April to the end of summer. Make sure strawberries are not white at the top part under the leaf and are not larger than normal. Fresh aroma is another good sign. They stay fresh for three days in the refrigerator.

Watermelon: A whole watermelon stays fresh for a week. Once it is cut and sliced, it is only fresh for a day in the refrigerator.

WHAT KIND OF CONTAINERS KEEP FOOD "FRESH AND NUTRITIOUS"?

Food containers come in metal, plastic, glass, and terracotta. The ideal food containers are so-called neutral ones, meaning the material does not interact chemically with the food. The interaction of a substance in the container with the food it touches or vice versa is an undesired effect. Mainly, glass containers are the healthiest. No substance in glass reacts with food, and the flavor of foods or liquids stored in glass is unchanged. However, colorless glass containers absorb light. When milk and yogurt, especially, are kept in glass containers under bright light, there can be some loss of B vitamin, which is sensitive to light. Food kept in the refrigerator has no significant loss of vitamins since the inside of the refrigerator is dark.

- Paper wraps are also good for storage. Various kinds of grease-resistant paper food wraps are suitable for deli, breakfast and meat products.
- Plastic containers are also very popular for storage. Since there are plastic containers in various qualities and types, look for ones that are approved by the Ministry of Health and a well-known brand. We do not recommend storing cooked food in plastic containers.
- Glazed terracotta containers are used to store products such as molasses, cheese, and yogurt. When subjected to heat, harmful substances in these containers such as lead, and cadmium can interact with the food. Therefore, we advise that you do not use them unless necessary.

HOW TO CUT AND SLICE FOOD

Should I use a knife to cut greens?

Cutting greens with a metal or steel knife increases the risk of oxidation, or browning around the cut edge, and loss of vitamins. The oxidation does not occur immediately after cutting. However, if the salad is to be eaten several hours later, it loses much of its vitamins within that period of time.

Should bamboo, plastic or ceramic knives be preferred?

It would be an exaggeration to say that bamboo, plastic or ceramic knives are healthier than the metal knives. Vitamin loss in food slows down when these knives are used, but it is not completely prevented. The knife should be sharp. Because these alternative knives are not sharp enough, they may smash the vegetables and fruits. Smashed vegetables, fruits, and greens may have more vitamin loss than normal.

Should we use a blender?

Using a blender to speed up food preparation is not recommended since it processes the food and increases the acid level. Whipping, mixing, or mashing the food with normal methods is always the healthiest.

THINGS TO KNOW ABOUT VEGETABLES

How should fresh vegetables be cooked?

You should cook your vegetable in the shortest time possible and with the least amount of water, or steam it. Cook fresh spinach, broccoli, cauliflower, cabbage, okra, eggplant, and zucchini as quickly as possible. For fresh green beans, 20 minutes is enough for cooking. Do not add ingredients such as soda water or bicarbonate. Such ingredients cause the loss of A, B and C vitamins.

Make your salad healthy and tasty

It is necessary to pay attention to several tips when preparing the salad to make it as delicious as it is nutritious. Do not skip these details while preparing a salad:

- Do not use wet ingredients. Wet ingredients prevent the salad dressing from being absorbed.

- Since the oil keeps the salt from dissolving, add it last.

- To distribute the salad dressing evenly, first mix it well in a separate cup and then drizzle it over the salad.

- Instead of cutting romaine and iceberg lettuce with a metal knife, you can choose to slice it with a wooden knife or tear it by hand.

- Add potato salad dressing when the potatoes are warm so that the dressing is absorbed completely.

Washing vegetables

One of the most important rules you need to take into consideration when you prepare your vegetables for cooking is to first wash them and then peel or cut them. If you let your vegetables sit out after cleaning them, there will be a loss of vitamin C. For root vegetables, first separate the root part from green parts and then wash the vegetable. Washing vegetables should be done prior to slicing them. The most hygienic and correct way is to wash them one by one under running water. Soaking vegetables in water or in a water-vinegar mixture does not make them more hygienic. Vinegar does not remove pesticides on the vegetables. Only greens should be washed in a water-vinegar mixture for disinfection. The best way to wash leafy vegetables is the pool method, done by transferring vegetables from one bowl to another.

Preparing the vegetables

Use your hands as much as possible to prepare your vegetables. Using knives or other blades may cause a change in the texture of your vegetables.

Storage life of vegetables

To ensure high nutritional value, cook vegetables immediately after buying them without delay. If you cannot cook them immediately, store in accordance with the most appropriate storing conditions.

Cutting the vegetables

To avoid loss of nutritional value in vegetables, they should first be washed, then be prepared and later cut. Making the cutting process the last step before cooking can help prevent the loss of vitamins and minerals in vegetables.

Extending the life of vegetables

Storing vegetables by freezing is a healthy method that maintains peak nutritional value. Still, eating natural foods, consuming them seasonally and fresh should be your priority. If you must, you can store vegetables in the freezer after blanching them by cooking briefly in boiling water. By plunging the tender-crisp vegetables and fruits in the cold water, you can stop the cooking. After this process, you can freeze and store them for a while longer.

Since defrosting frozen food in hot water may increase the growth of bacteria, it is not recommended. If you have no other alternative, then use cold water and change the water every half-hour.

> **Prepare delicious vegetable dishes with their vibrant colors!**
>
> People tend to have two main complaints about vegetable dishes: the strong smell of some food leaching in the dish and green vegetables losing their color. There is one simple solution for both of these issues. Keep the lid slightly open while cooking food with strong smells such as onion, cauliflower, and cabbage. Keeping the lid slightly open as you cook the green vegetables will allow steam to escape, and that will prevent green vegetables from losing color. If you do not want your vegetables to lose color, you can add a little vinegar to the water while cooking.

Practical hints

- To prevent apples from spoiling in the fridge, do not let them touch one another and keep the stem parts upright.
- Wet your knife in hot water to prevent your hard-boiled egg from smearing. Do not dry your knife before slicing the egg.
- You can use the same method for slicing fresh bread, but this time dry the knife immediately after soaking it in hot water. With this method, you will be able to cut the bread without wrecking the loaf.
- You should toss dried fruits and nuts in flour to prevent them from sinking to the bottom when you make a cake with those ingredients. You will see that coating with flour helps them distribute evenly throughout the batter.
- Put a cup of water under the grill to avoid smoke when you have a barbecue at home. Water absorbs both the smoke and the oil.

HYGIENE IN THE KITCHEN

One of the important steps in eating healthy is to prepare and store food in a hygienic environment. I recommend the following precautions in the kitchen to prevent contamination, what I call "environmental pollution."

Cutting boards: The knife marks that eventually occur on a cutting board run the risk of harboring bacteria. Use a separate cutting board for fresh produce, another board for raw meat, chicken, and fish, and a different board for ready-to-eat foods (like bread). In this way, contamination of uncooked food items, such as a salad, from raw meat is prevented.

Cleaning the stove and oven: Food crumbs and oils frequently get stuck in stoves and ovens. Clean up those food and oil remains without delay.

Countertops: Hygiene is very important when it comes to kitchen counters, which are constantly in contact with water and food. It is necessary to wipe down the countertop regularly to keep it clean.

Kitchen sinks: Do not put food waste and liquids such as oil and tea down the sink. Be careful to keep it clean at all times.

Wash out the trash cans: Trash cans cultivate bacteria quickly. Empty your trash can as often as possible and use it again only after cleaning it with bleach.

Sponges and kitchen towels: Wet and humid environments are ideal for the growth of bacteria. Sponges and kitchen towels also carry risk of contamination. Therefore, they should frequently be sterilized.

Do not forget these

- There's no need to avoid oils or fats. We should consume oils or fats as naturally as possible, as we consume other foods.
- Oils are sensitive to heat. You should consume oils in their natural state without allowing any formation of trans fats.
- Our body does not produce Omega 3 or Omega 6 fats. We need to get them from foods that are rich in them, as both help to maintain a comfortable pregnancy as well as to promote the neurodevelopment of the baby.
- Olive oil is of great value, but be careful to use oil without over-heating it. Choose an olive oil produced by traditional methods.

THINGS YOU NEED TO CONSIDER IN YOUR NUTRITION

1. It's important to drink 8 to 10 glasses of water each day.
2. You can drink a maximum of 2 cups of herbal and fruit teas such as black tea, linden, rose hip, or apple, brewed for 3 to 4 minutes, every day.
3. Make sure that the fruits and vegetables you consume are seasonal, organic and chemical-free.
4. Use olive oil in your meals and try not to burn it while cooking.
5. Use plenty of onions and garlic in your meals.

6. To increase the nutritional value of your soups and meals, use lean bone broth.
7. Limit your daily consumption of salt to 5 grams, and use iodized salt.
8. Arrange your eating schedule to be sure you have your breakfast within 30 minutes after you get up.
9. Finish your night snack two hours before you go to bed.
10. Do not consume alcoholic and caffeinated beverages like strong tea, coffee, and cola.
11. Stay away from sugar and artificial sweeteners.
12. Do not consume processed foods (all kinds of pre-packaged products).

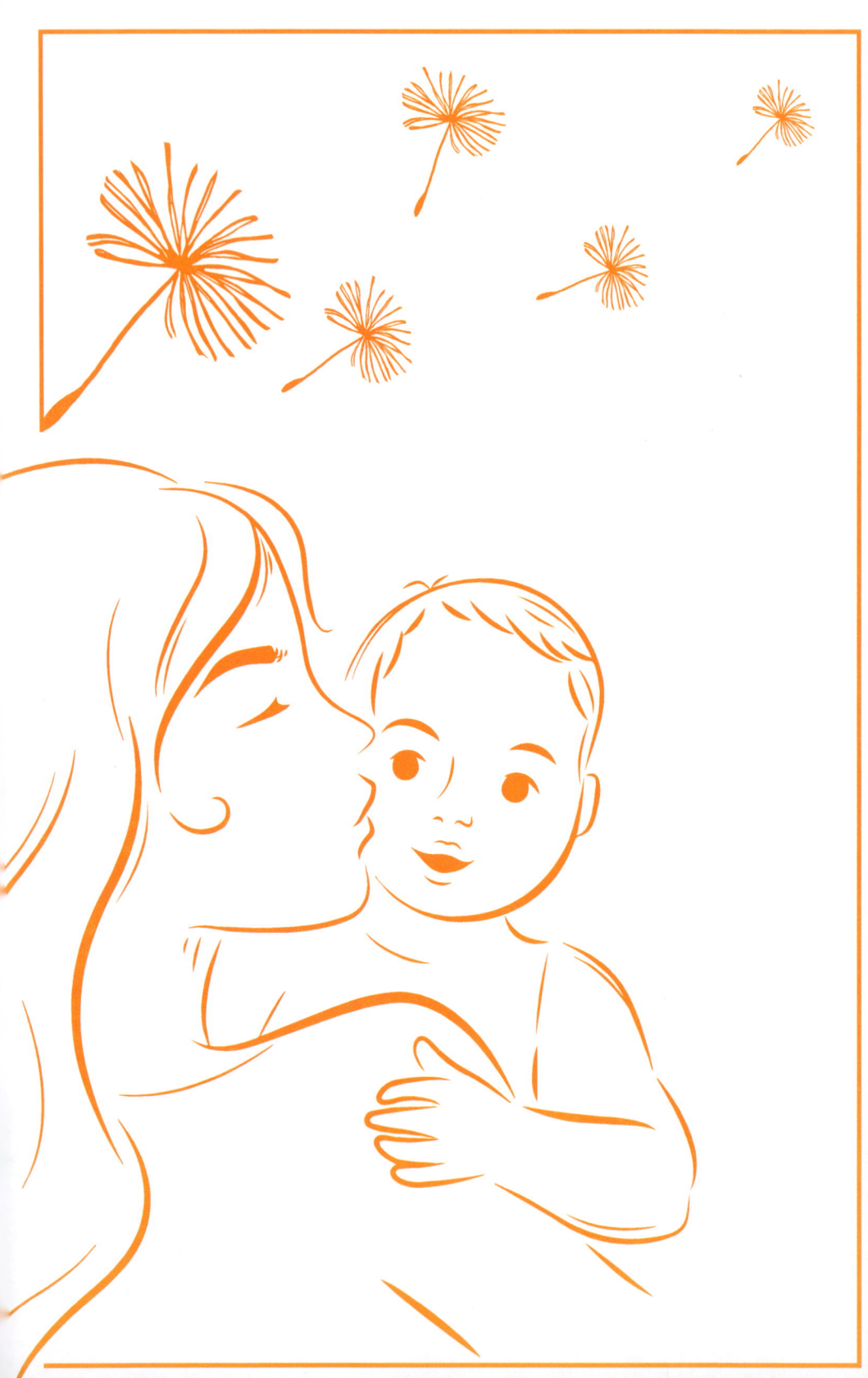

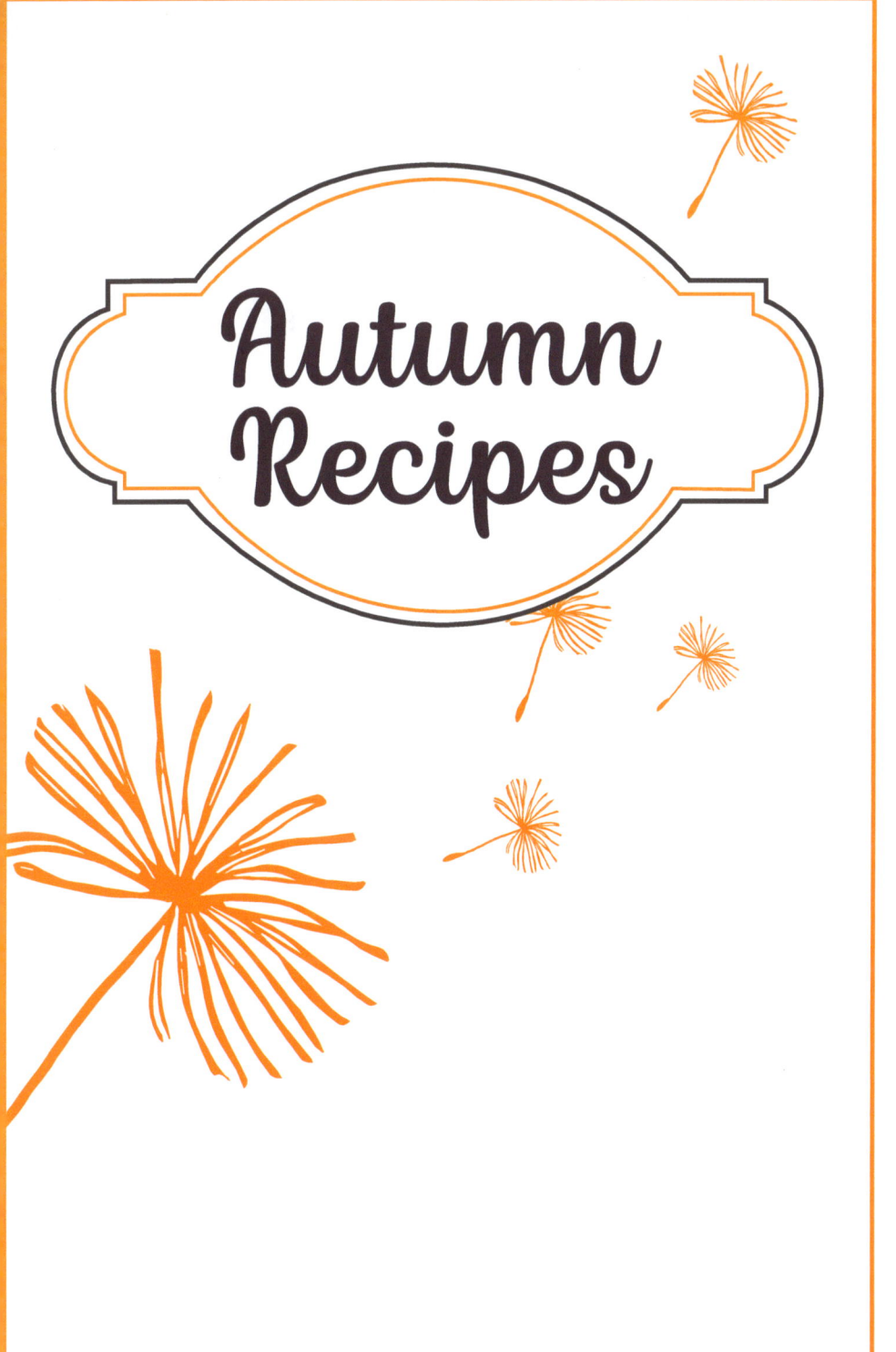

Tomato Soup

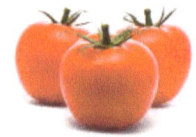

MAKES 4-6 SERVINGS

Ingredients

- 5 Tomatoes
- 1 Teaspoon Organic Whole Wheat Flour
- 4-5 Tablespoon Coconut Oil
- 1 Liter Hot Water
- Salt
- Goat Cheese

Directions

1. Finely chop the tomatoes.
2. Melt the coconut oil in the pan.
3. Stir in the flour and cook until medium brown.
4. Whisk in the tomatoes and stir constantly as you cook for 10 minutes.
5. Gradually add the hot water, let it come to a boil.
6. Season with salt to taste before turning the heat off.
7. Serve in soup bowls and sprinkle the crumbled goat cheese on top.

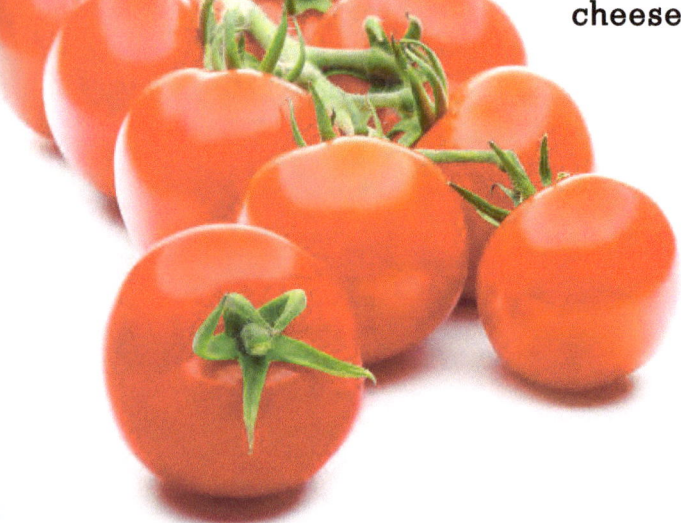

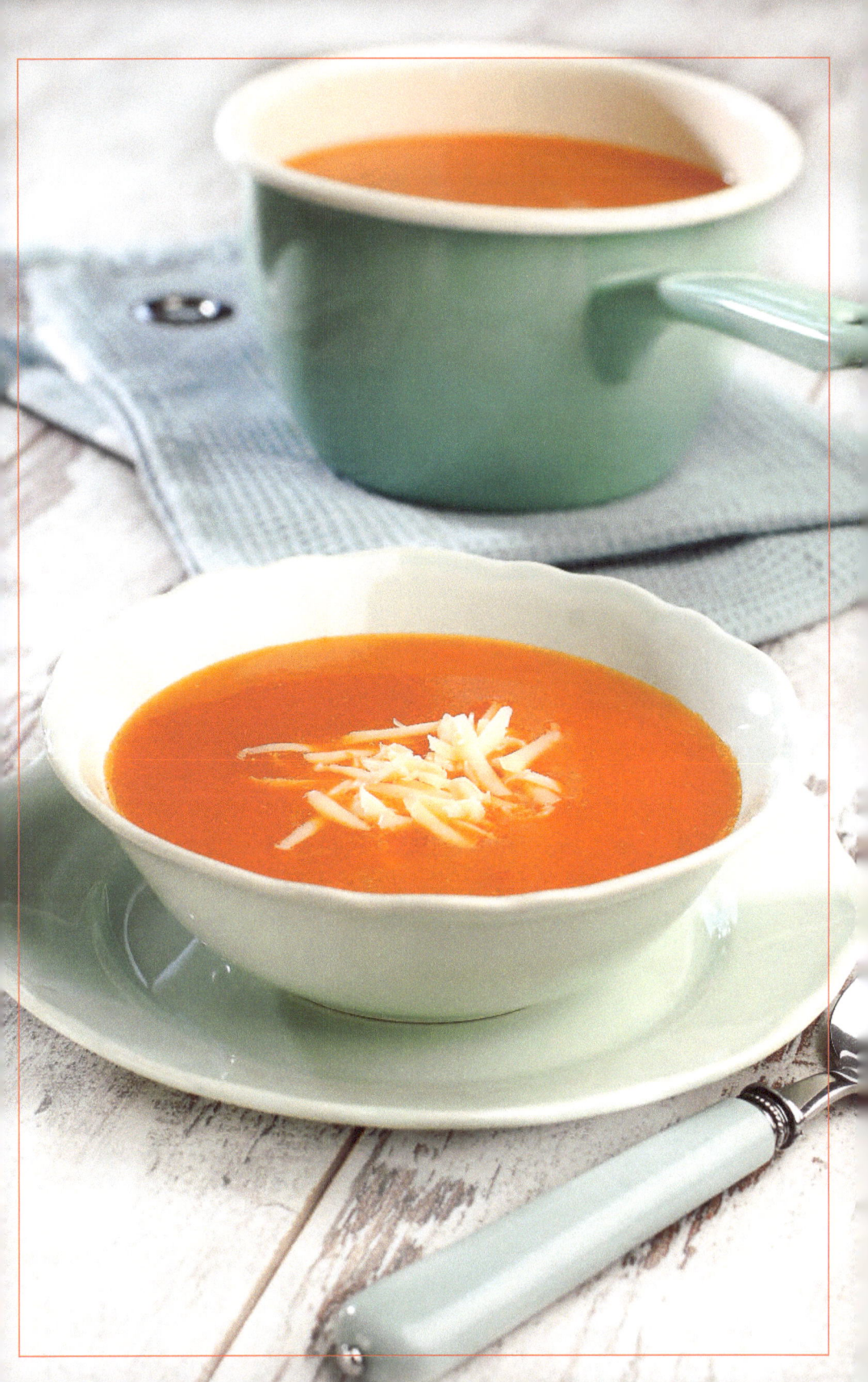

Brown Rice Salad

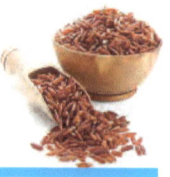

MAKES 4-6 SERVINGS

Ingredients

- 200ml Brown Rice
- 200ml Water
- 65ml Cold Water
- 1 Onion
- 1 Zucchini
- Olive Oil
- Salt
- 1 Carrot
- 1 Pinch Mediterranean Greens
- Raisin, Pumpkin Seed, Sunflower Seed

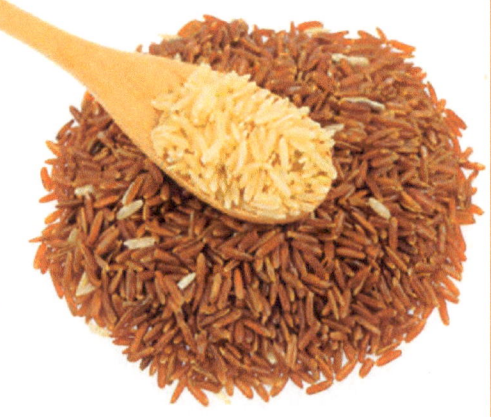

Directions

1. Peel the skin off the onion, dice the onion into medium pieces and the zucchini into thin slices.
2. In a pot, add the olive oil and heat it slightly.
3. Add onion and zucchini, stirring continually, and cook on medium heat.
4. Season with salt.
5. Add the pre-washed brown rice and 200ml water, cover the pot and let it simmer.
6. Before the water totally boils down, add the cold water and bring back to a simmer until all the water is boiled down.
7. Transfer to a large bowl.
8. Mince the greens and grate the carrot.
9. Add raisins, pumpkin seeds, and sunflower seeds.
10. Add a little more olive oil, if desired.
11. Serve warm.

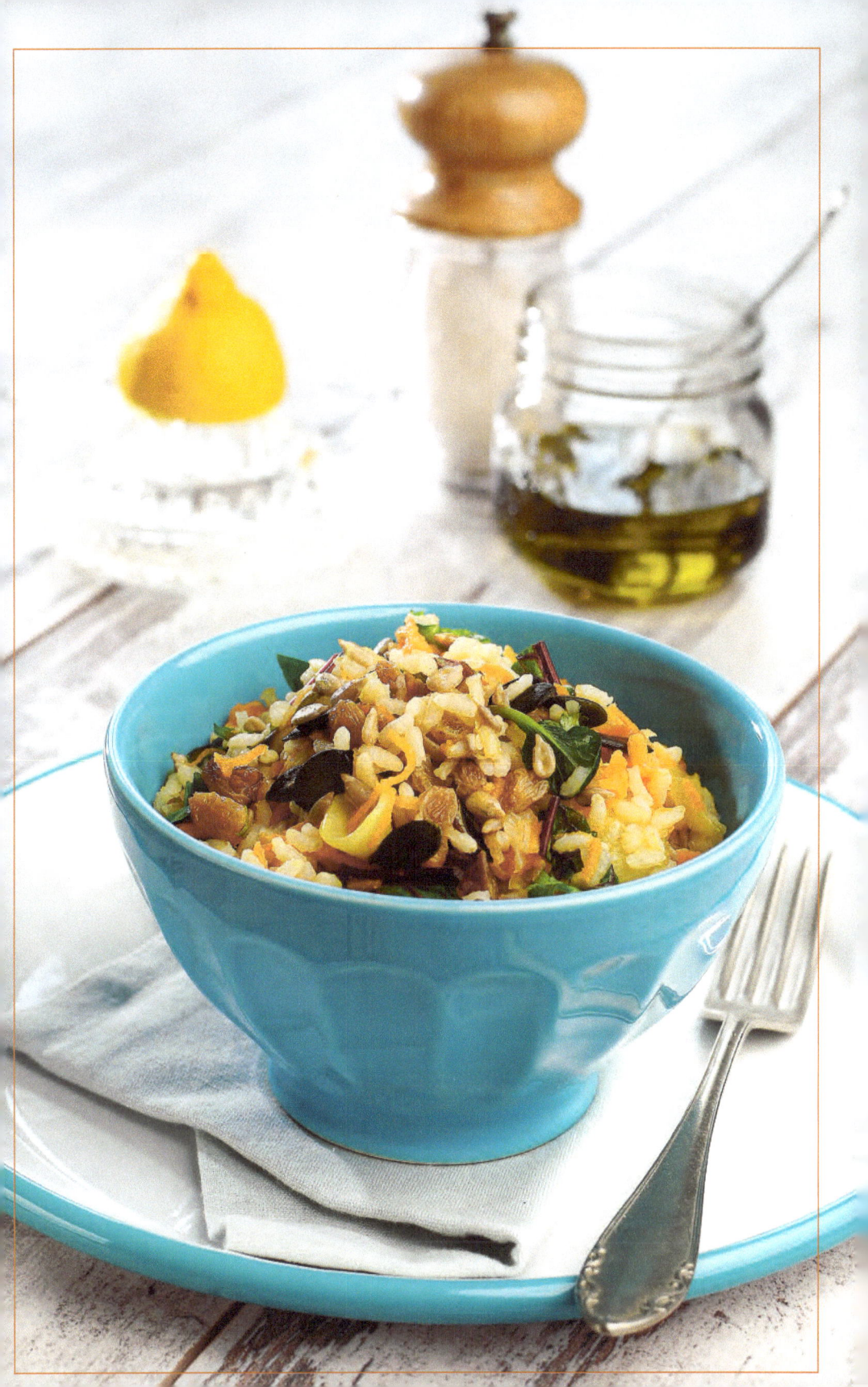

Oven Baked Fish

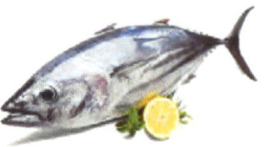

MAKES 2 SERVINGS

Ingredients

- 1 Large Sea Bream
- 1 Large Onion
- 1-2 SM Potatoes
- 1-2 SM Carrots
- 4-5 Garlic Cloves
- Sea Salt
- 1-2 Bay Leaves
- Olive Oil
- Several Sprigs Rosemary and Fresh Thyme
- Black Pepper

Directions

1. Clean the fish and wash it.
2. Chop the garlic into large pieces and mix with olive oi and salt.
3. Season the fish inside and on top with the above mixture.
4. Stuff the bay leaves, rosemary and thyme into the cavity.
5. Let sit in the refrigerator for 40 minutes.
6. Slice the onions and place them in the bottom of the baking dish.
7. In the same way, place the carrots and the potatoes.
8. Place the fish over the onions.
9. Bake it in preheated oven at 190C.

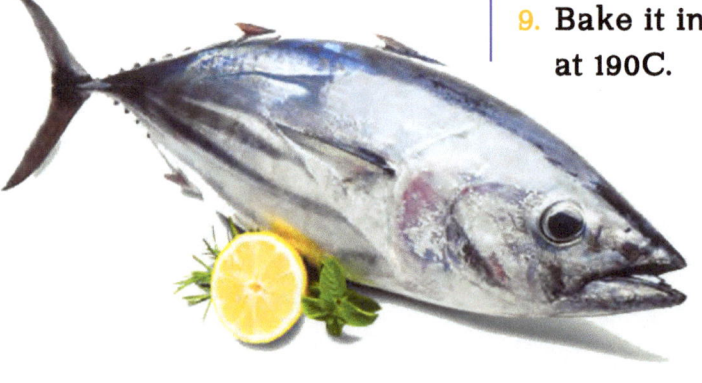

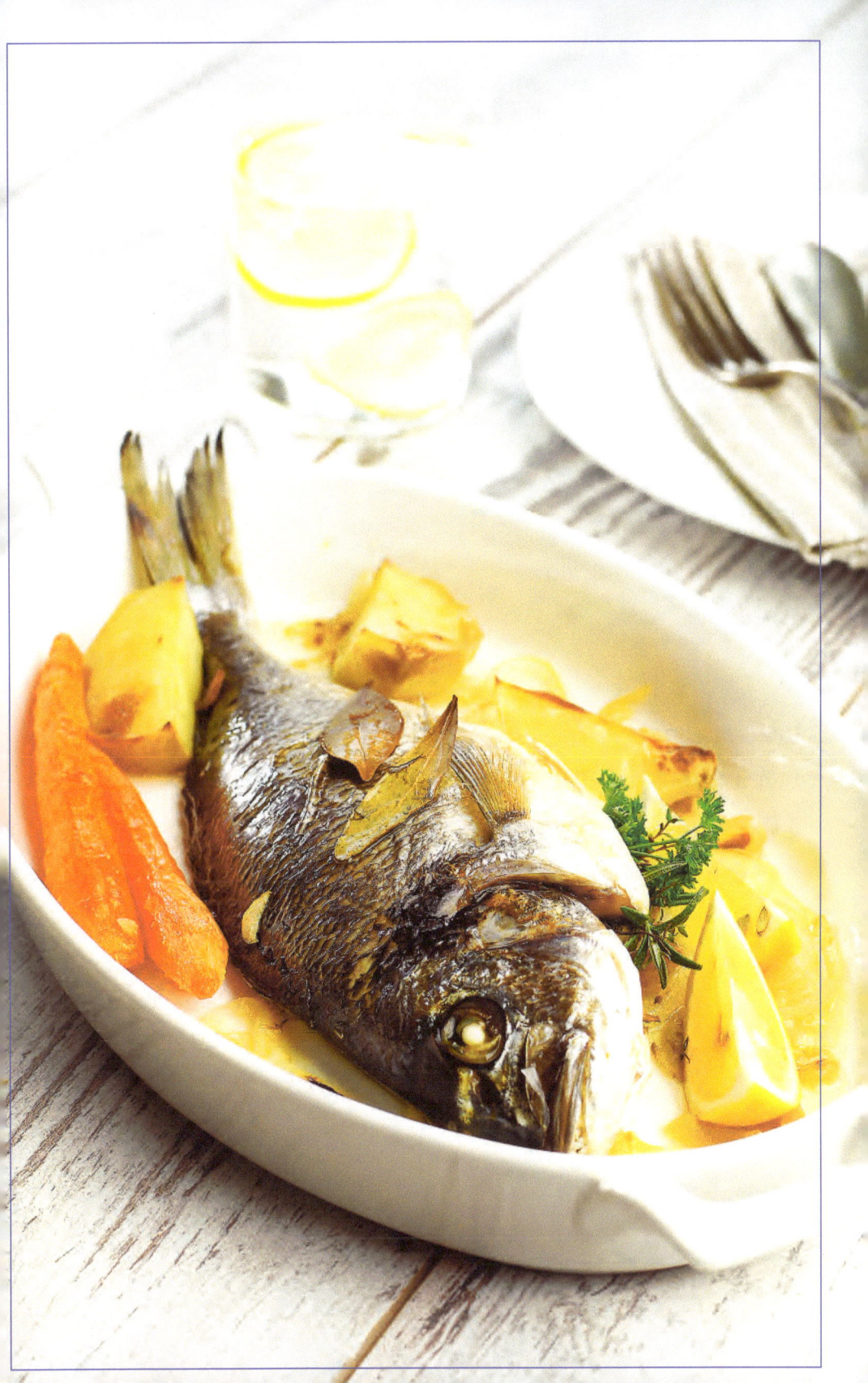

No Bake Carrot Cake

MAKES 7-8 SERVINGS

Ingredients

- 3 Medium Carrots
- 200g Oats
- 150g Dates
- 4-5 Dried Figs
- 100ml Raw Almonds
- 2 Teaspoon Cinnamon Powder

For the Frosting

- 180g Cashews
- 140ml Coconut Milk
- 5 Dates
- ½ Vanilla Bean
- Walnuts and Orange Peel, for Garnish

Directions

1. Soak cashews in water for 3-4 hours.
2. If you have a power blender, add all the cake ingredients to the blender and blend until it becomes a coarse, sticky mix. If you don't have a power blender, grate the carrots first and then add to the blender with other ingredients.
3. Put the mixture into a 20x20cm cake pan.
4. Drain the cashews and add to the blender with frosting ingredients.
5. Blend until creamy, then spread the frosting evenly to coat the carrot cake.
6. Garnish with crumbled walnuts and add orange peel on top.

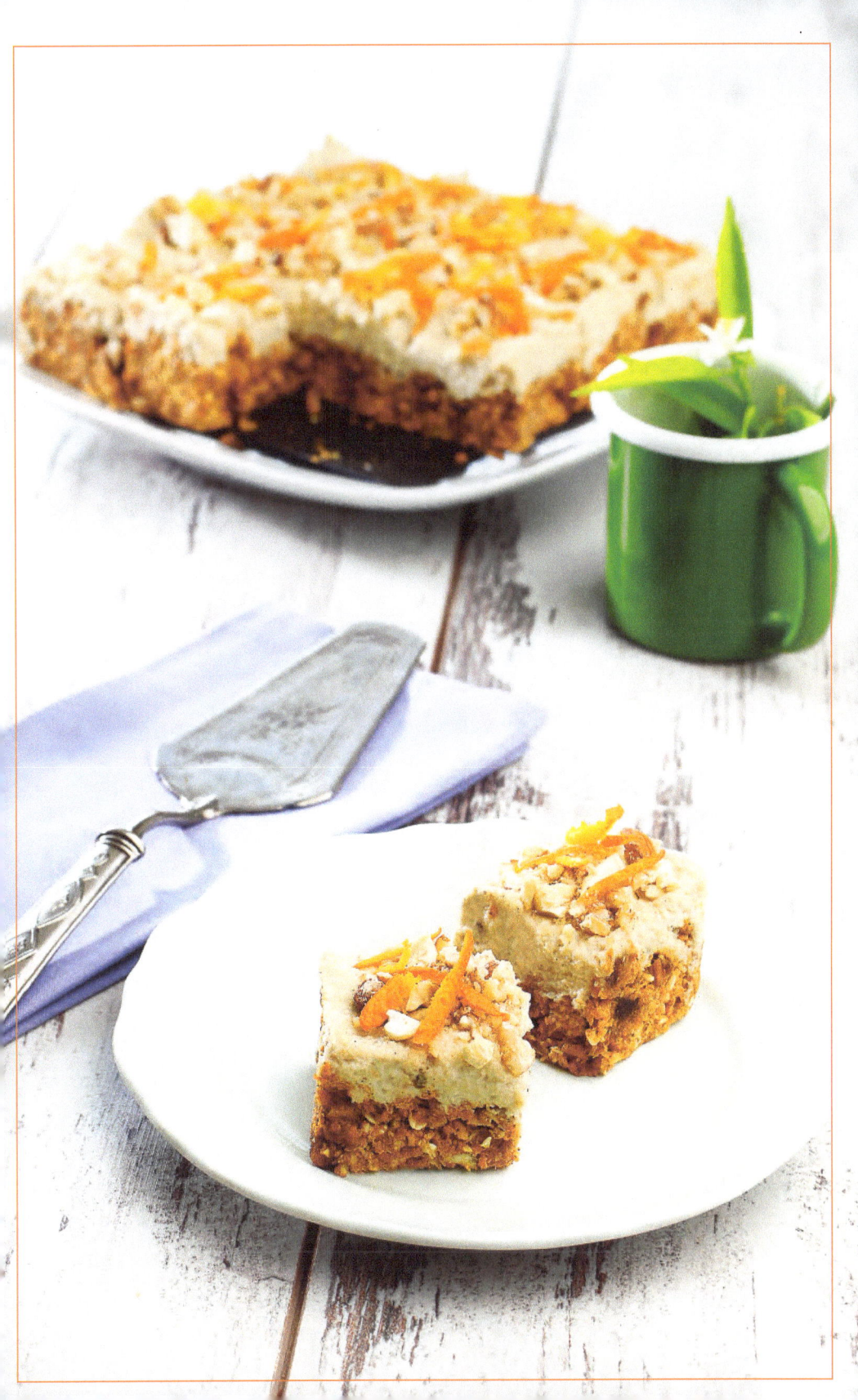

Flaxseed Cracker

MAKES 10 SERVINGS

Ingredients

- 400ml Flaxseed
- 200ml Water
- 2 Dessertspoons Cinnamon Powder
- 8-10 Cardamom Pods
- 1 Tablespoon Chia Seeds
- 1 TablespoonSunflower Seed Kernels
- 1 Tablespoon Sesame Seeds

Directions

1. Wash and drain the flax seeds, add 200ml water and mix in the cinnamon powder and ground cardamom.
2. Cover and store in the refridgerator overnight.
3. Spread the flax seed mixture evenly on a sheet of parchment paper, cover with another sheet of parchment paper, and roll it out into a 3-4 mm layer with a rolling pin.
4. Remove the top sheet of parchment paper and slice the flat flax seed mixture into the desired cracker size.
5. Sprinkle sunflower kernels, chia seeds and sesame seeds over the slices.
6. Transfer the parchment paper and unbaked crackers to a flat baking tray.
7. Bake at 180C for an hour.
8. Flip the crackers over with a spatula to make sure each is crispy and all moisture is gone (note: they'll go moldy if there's any moisture left).
9. Crackers can be stored in the refridgerator for months if completely dry.
10. You can eat these crackers between meals—dip them in coconut or almond milk, or top with grated apple or pear for breakfast.

These crackers are a rich source of Omega 3. Enjoy!

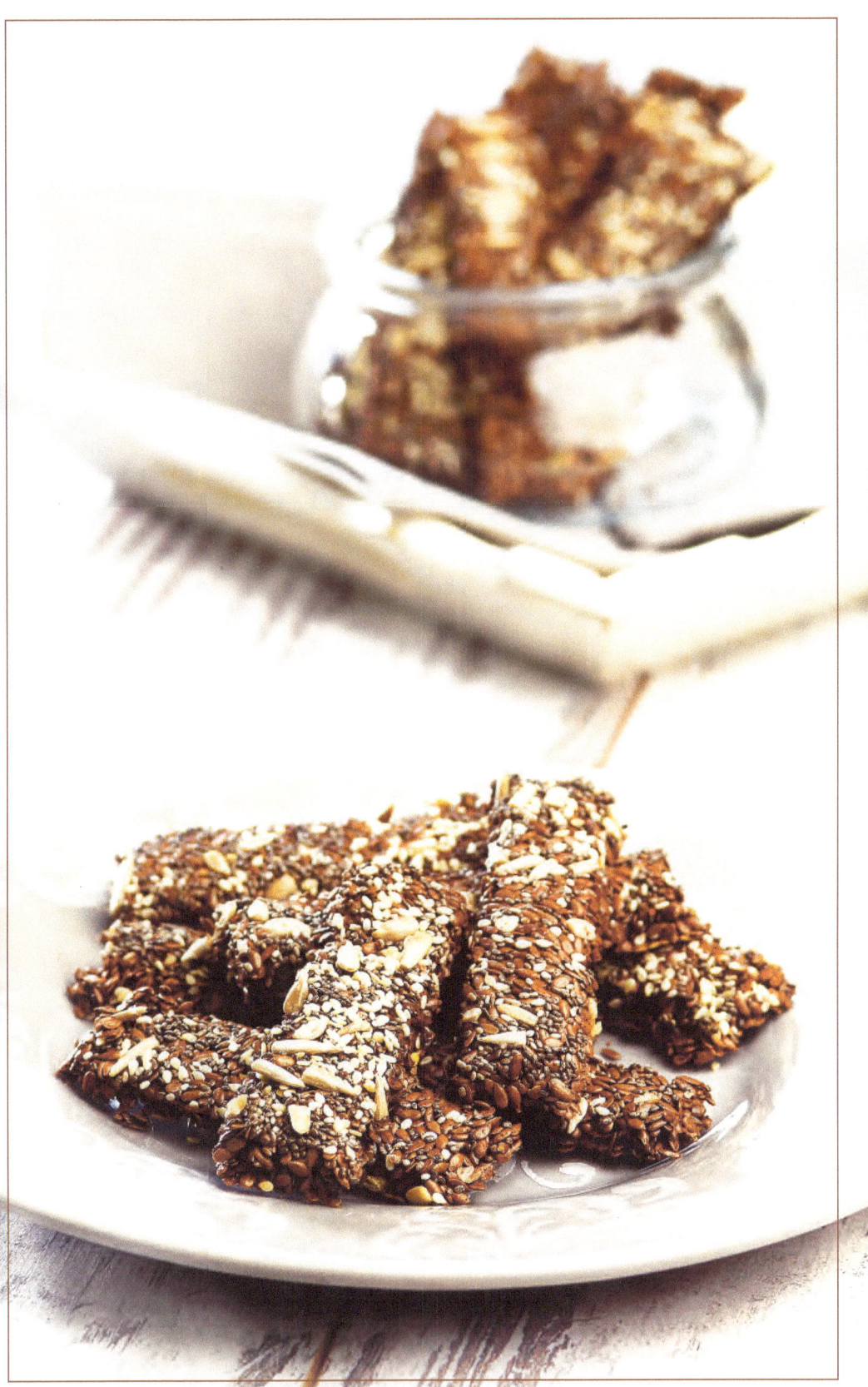

Maca-Banana Smoothie

MAKES 2 SERVINGS

Ingredients

- 400ml Coconut Milk
- 2 Bananas (preferably from Anamur)
- 5-6 Dates
- 2 Teaspoons Maca Powder

Directions

1. Remove seeds from the dates, peel the bananas.
2. Add coconut milk, bananas, dates, and maca powder into the blender and blend until smooth.
3. Pour into glasses to serve.

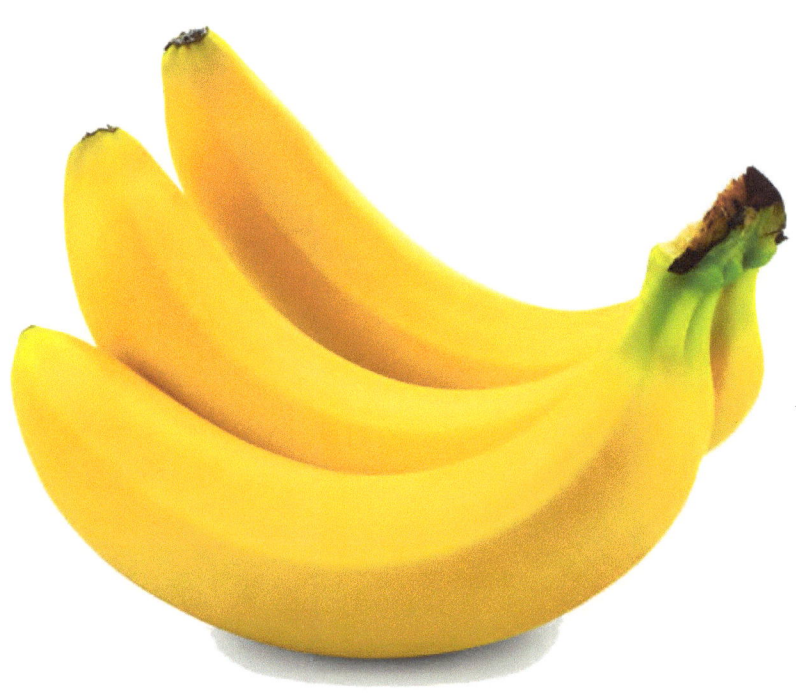

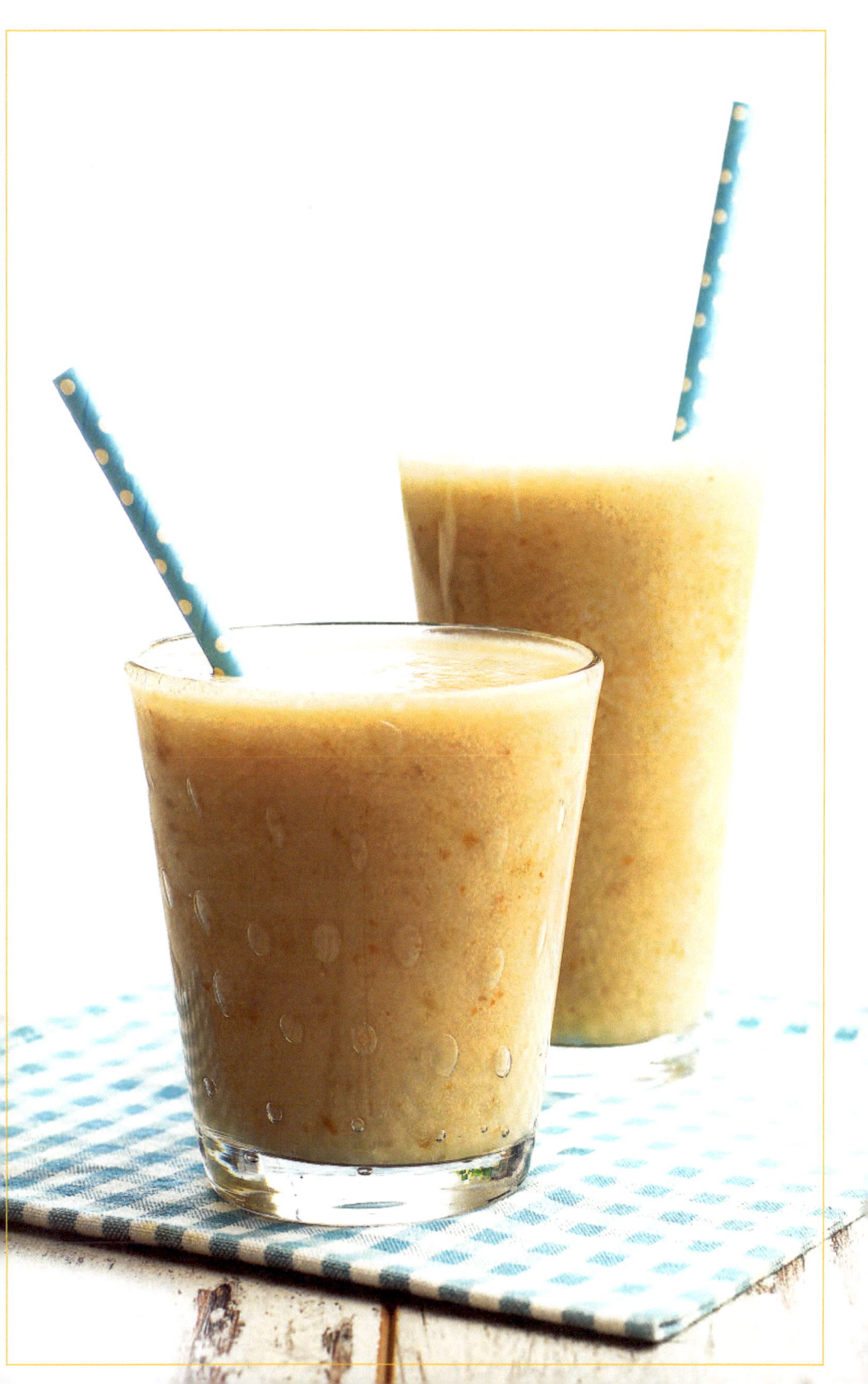

Tavern Style Siyez Wheat Bulgar Pilaf

MAKES 4 SERVINGS

Ingredients

- 200ml Siyez Wheat Bulgur (Einkorn Bulgur)
- 265ml Water
- 1 Onion
- 1 Large Tomato
- 3-4 Green Long Peppers
- Pinch of Fresh Mint, minced
- 2-3 Tablespoon Coconut Oil
- Salt

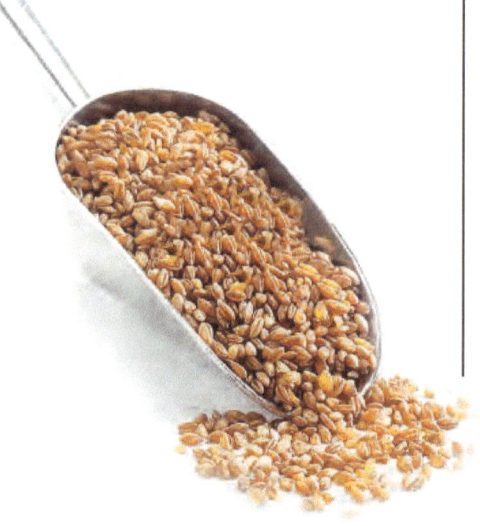

Directions

1. Peel the onion and slice it thinly.
2. Remove the seeds of the green peppers and cut into small pieces.
3. Finely chop the tomato.
4. Put the coconut oil in a pot.
5. Add onion and pepper and cook over medium heat.
6. Add the tomato and continually stir.
7. Add Siyez (Einkorn) wheat bulgur and the water, stir well.
8. Season with salt and simmer on low heat.
9. Spread the minced fresh mint on top when the pilaf is almost ready.
10. Put the lid back on and let it cool for 5 minutes before serving.

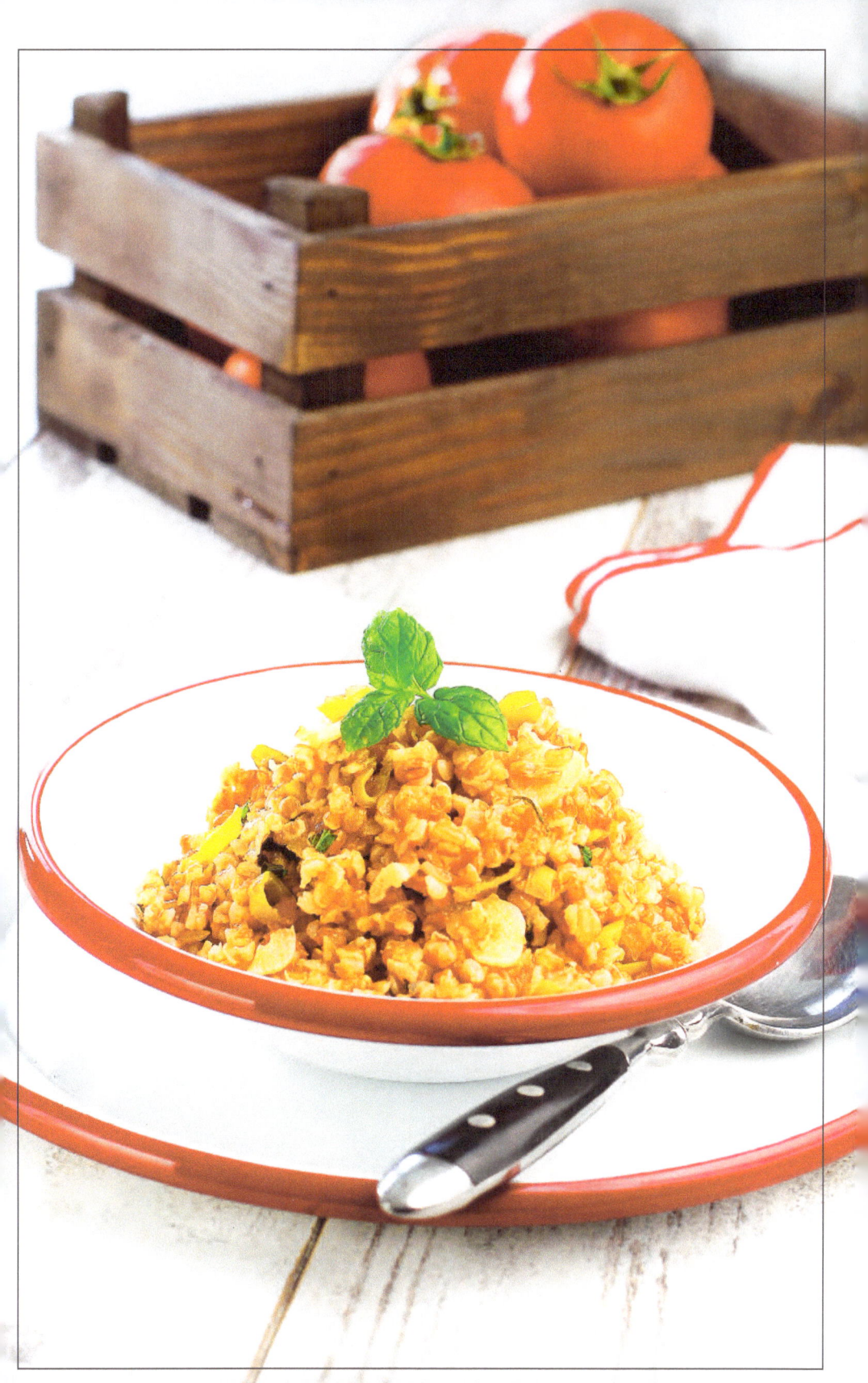

Celery Root with Leek Cooked with Olive Oil

MAKES 4-5 SERVINGS

Ingredients

- 3 Celery Roots
- 2 Leeks
- 1 Onion
- 1 Carrot
- 400ml Water
- 1 Lemon
- Olive Oil
- Salt

Directions

1. Slice the onion, cook in a little water and olive oil until the onions are tender.
2. Add the vegetables and the water.
3. Add a 100ml of olive oil before turning the heat off.
4. Season with salt.

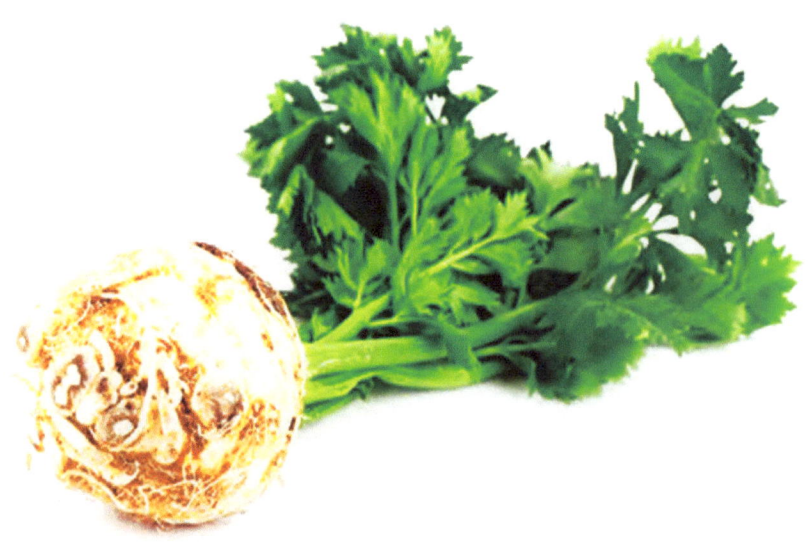

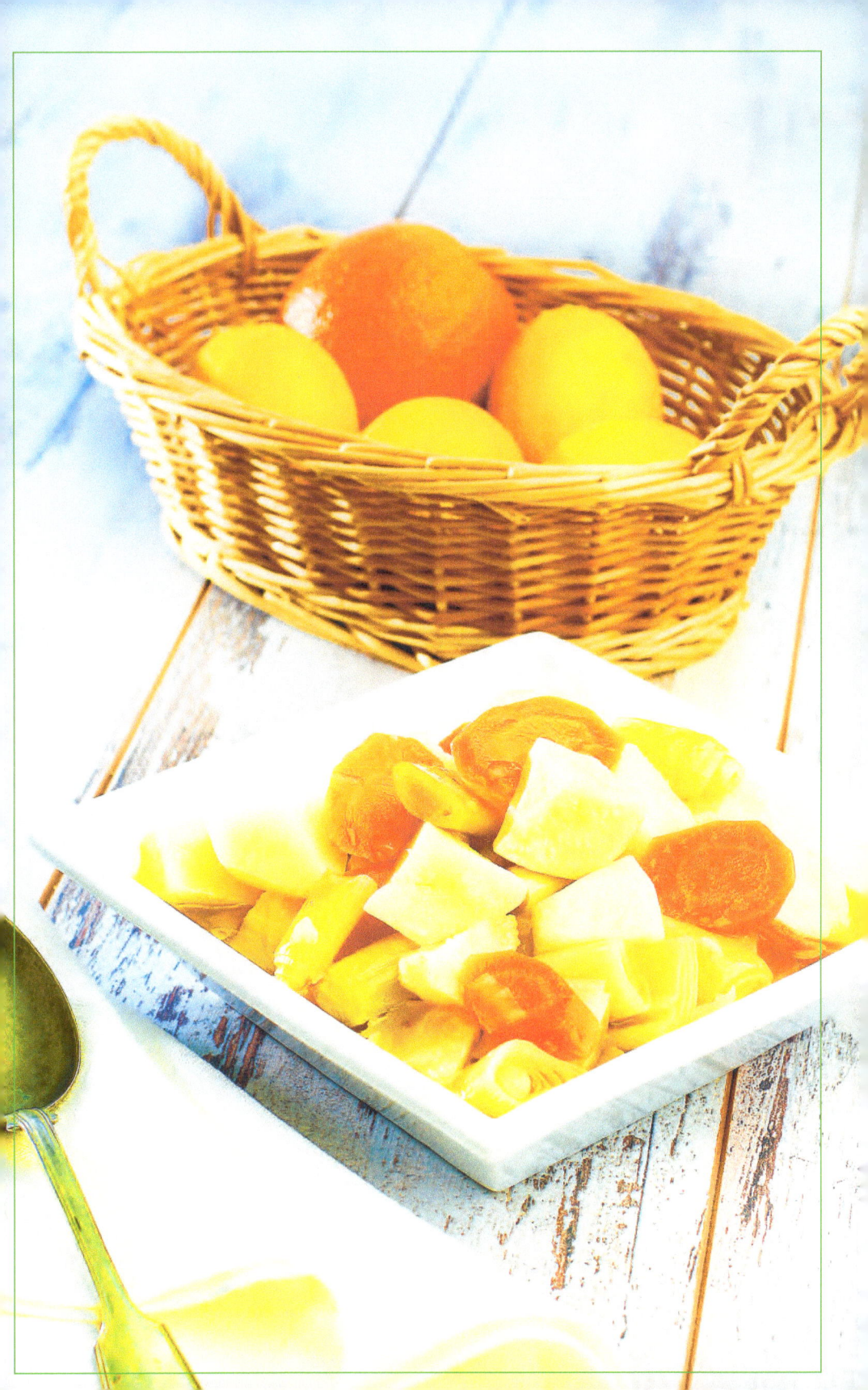

Omelet with Leek

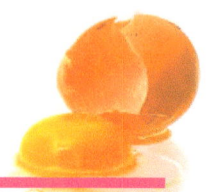

MAKES 1-2 SERVINGS

Ingredients

- 1 Leek
- 1 Carrot
- 1 Tablespoon Coconut Oil
- 2 Eggs
- 1 Tablespoon Goat Cheese
- 1 Pinch Nutmeg
- Salt

Directions

1. Melt coconut oil in a pan over medium heat.
2. Grate the carrot and thinly slice the leek, add to the pan and saute for 10 minutes until the vegetables are soft.
3. In a separate bowl, mix the eggs with goat cheese crumbles, salt, and nutmeg.
4. Pour the egg mixture over the leek and the carrot.
5. Cover the pan and cook for 5 more minutes.
6. Serve warm.

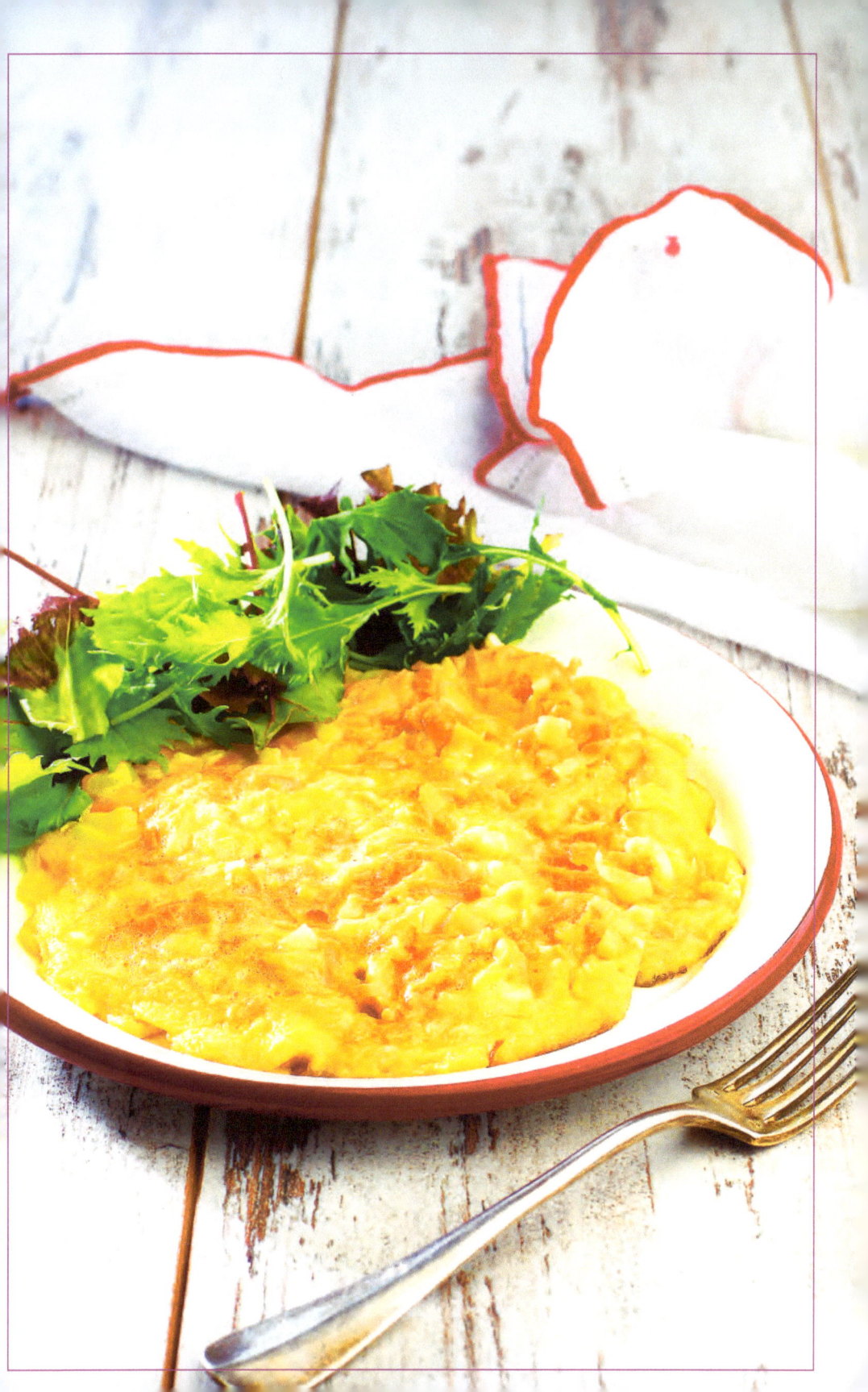

Palace Kofte

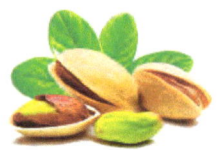

MAKES 6 SERVINGS

Ingredients

- 500g Ground Beef
- 1 Large Onion
- 4-5 Garlic Cloves
- 1 Egg
- 200ml Walnuts
- 100ml Pine Nut and Pistachio Mixture
- Cumin, Black Pepper, Sea Salt

Directions

1. Peel and thinly chop the garlic.
2. Grate the onion.
3. Finely chop the walnuts and other nuts.
4. Combine all the ingredients and knead well.
5. Let it sit in the refrigerator for an hour.
6. To shape your meatballs, take a large walnut-size portion of the mixture and roll into a ball.
7. Place meatballs on the baking pan and bake in a preheated oven at 180C for 25 to 30 minutes.
8. Serve hot.

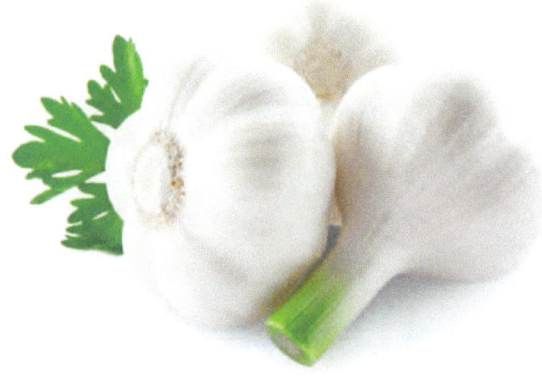

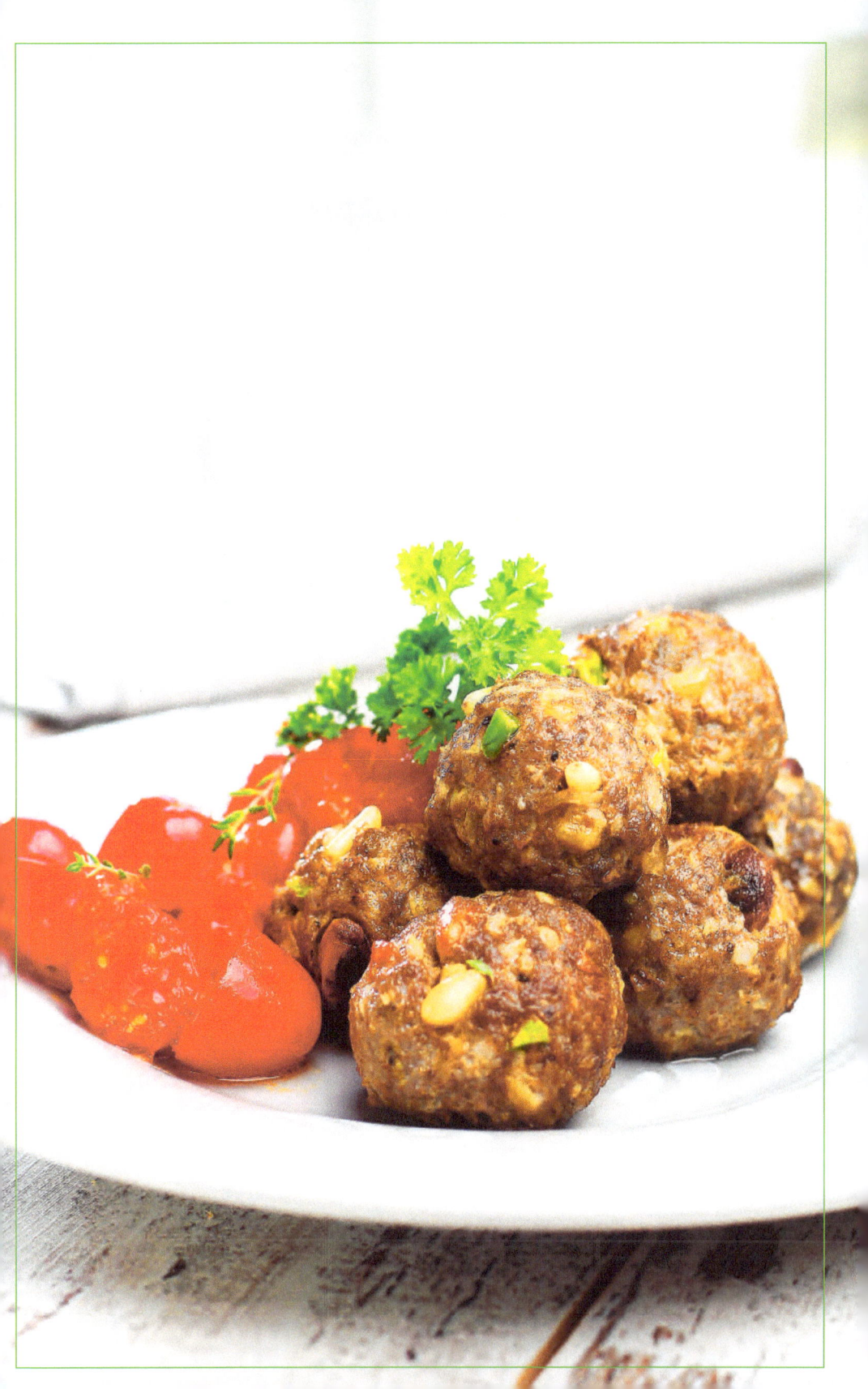

Beets with Garlic Yogurt

MAKES 4-5 SERVINGS

Ingredients

- 4-5 Medium Beets
- 1 Small Container Yogurt
- 3-4 Garlic Cloves, Mashed
- Salt
- Olive Oil

Directions

1. Peel, cut and boil the beets.
2. Add olive oil when warm and season with salt.
3. Let it cool and then serve with garlic yogurt.

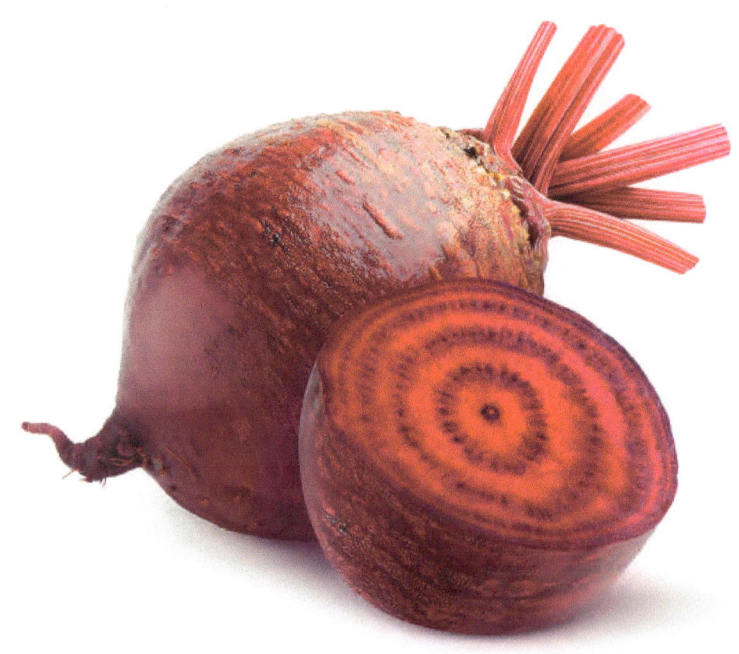

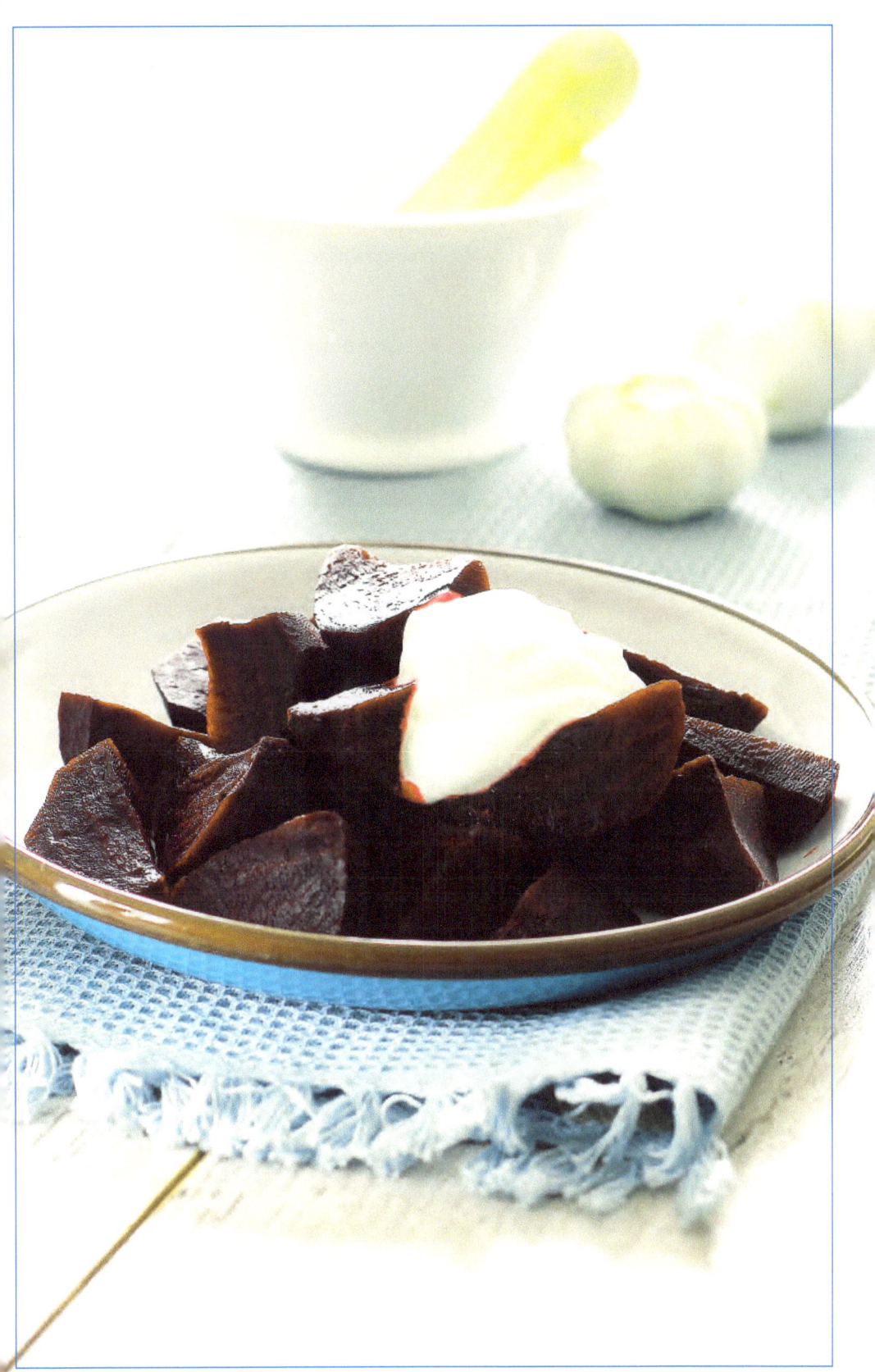

Sugar-Free Apple Jam

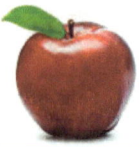

MAKES 4 SERVINGS

Ingredients

- 4 Apples
- 2 Apples for the Juice
- 1 Tablespoon Lemon Juice
- Cinnamon
- 2 Tablespoons Blanched Sliced Almonds

Directions

1. Grate apples and mix them in a pot with the apple juice.
2. Cook on medium heat.
3. Add the lemon juice when apples are soft.
4. Mix in a little cinnamon and blanched sliced almonds.
5. Pour into a jar when still hot and put on the lid.
6. Jam will stay fresh in the refrigerator for a week.

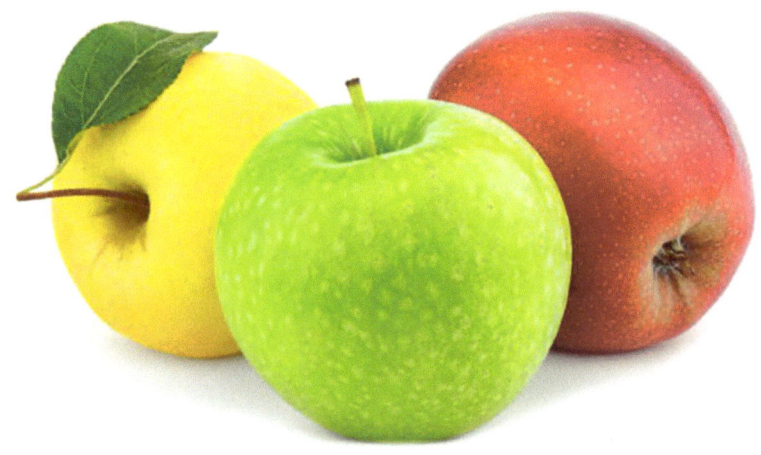

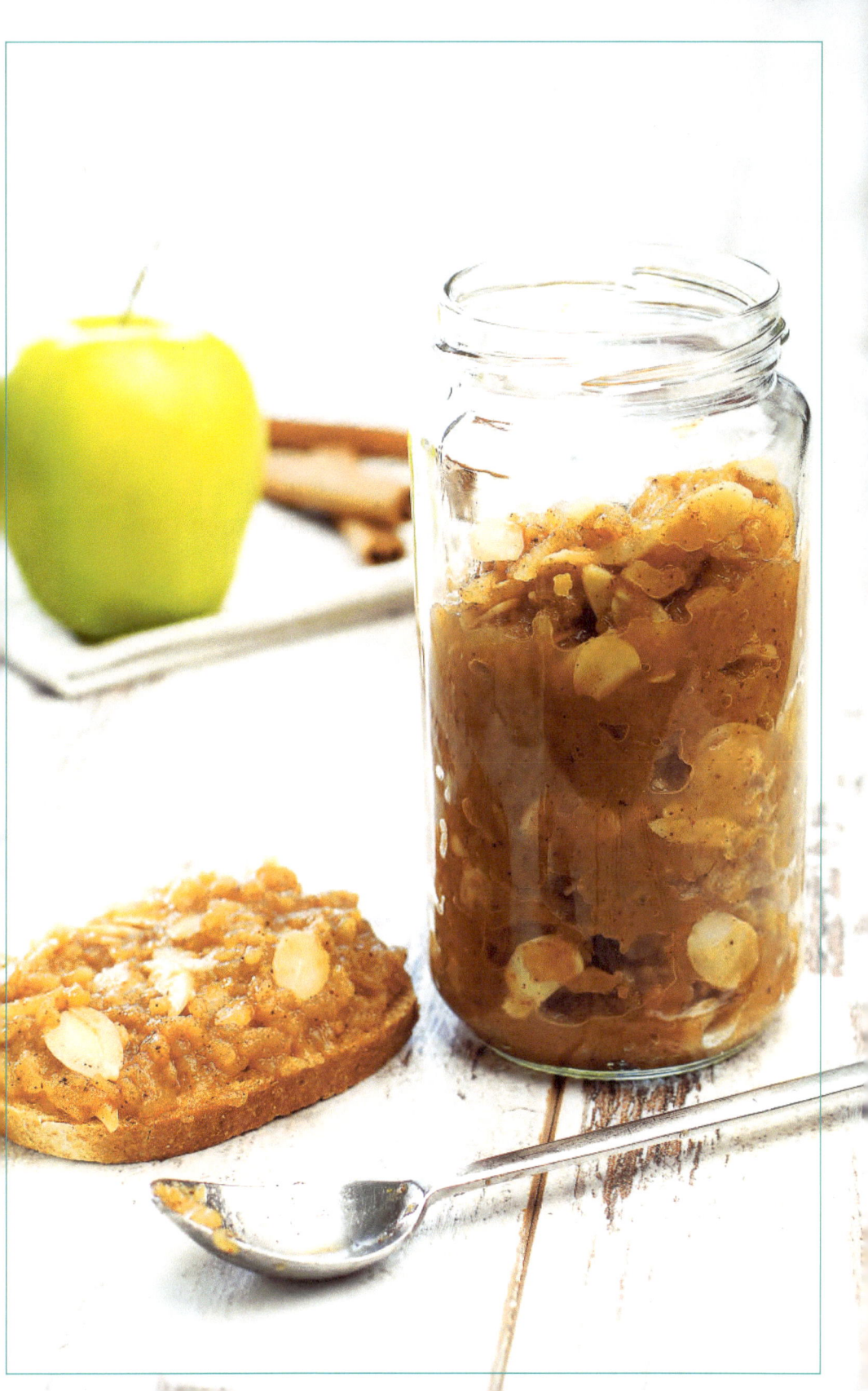

Sugar-Free Nut Cookies

MAKES 6-8 SERVINGS

Ingredients

- 400ml Organic Whole Wheat Flour
- 100g Butter (or Ghee)
- 4-5 Dried Apricots
- 2 Tablespoons Raisins
- 4-5 Dried Figs
- 2-3 Tablespoons Sunflower Seed Kernels
- 4-5 Walnuts, Coarsely Chopped

Directions

1. Soak dried fruits in hot water for a while, drain and rinse.
2. Mix all the ingredients and knead well.
3. Spread a sheet of parchment paper on a flat baking tray.
4. Take a large walnut-sized portion of the mixture, roll into a ball and place on the baking tray. Continue with the rest of the mixture.
5. Bake in the oven at 180C until brown.

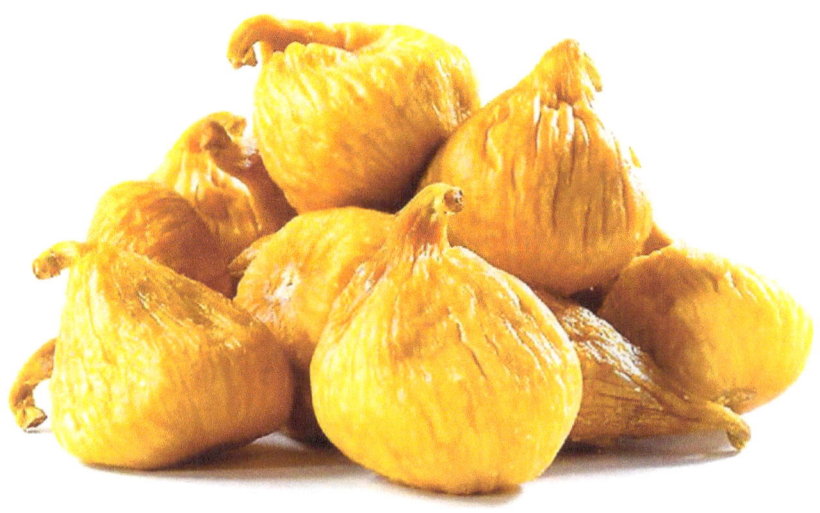

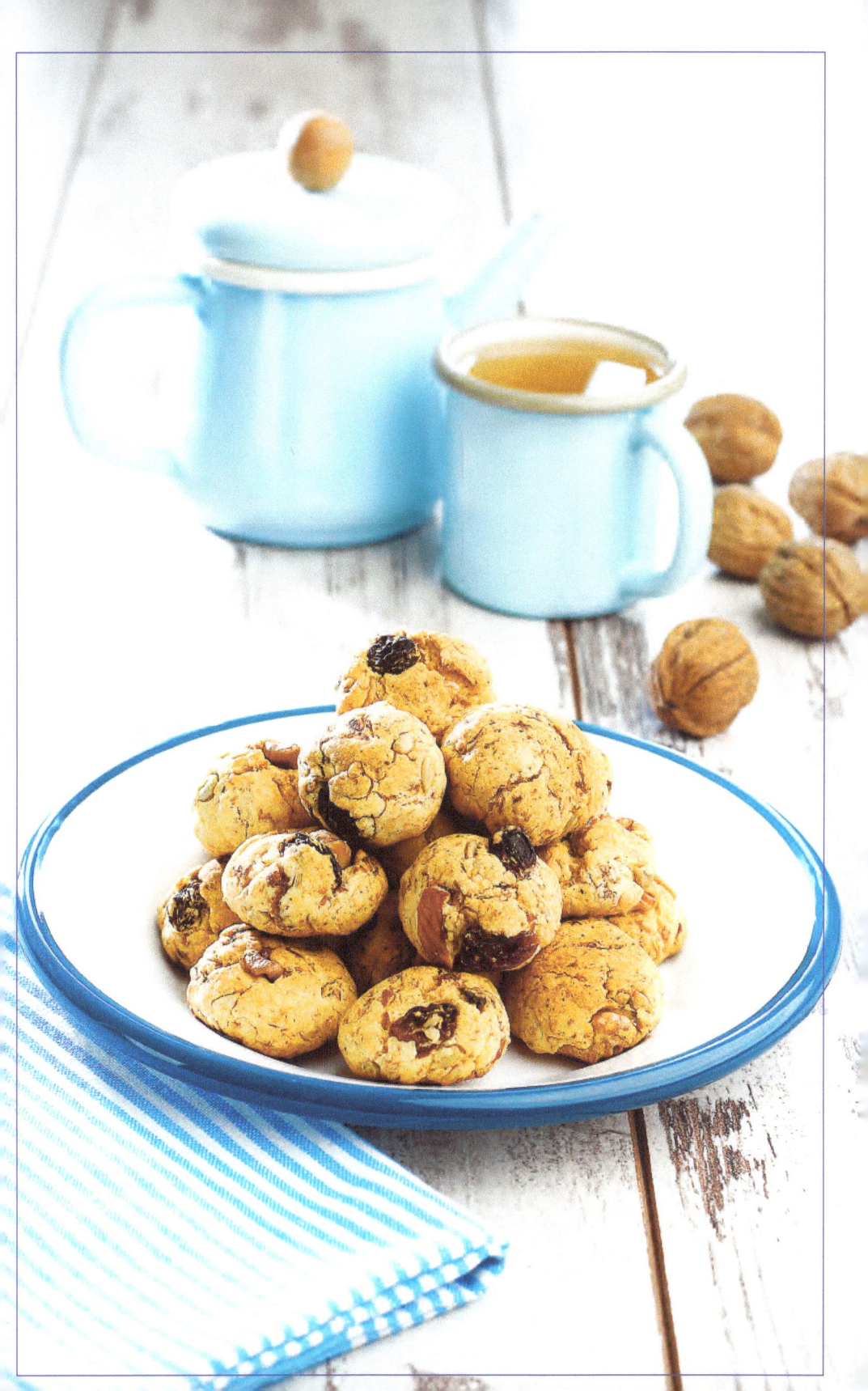

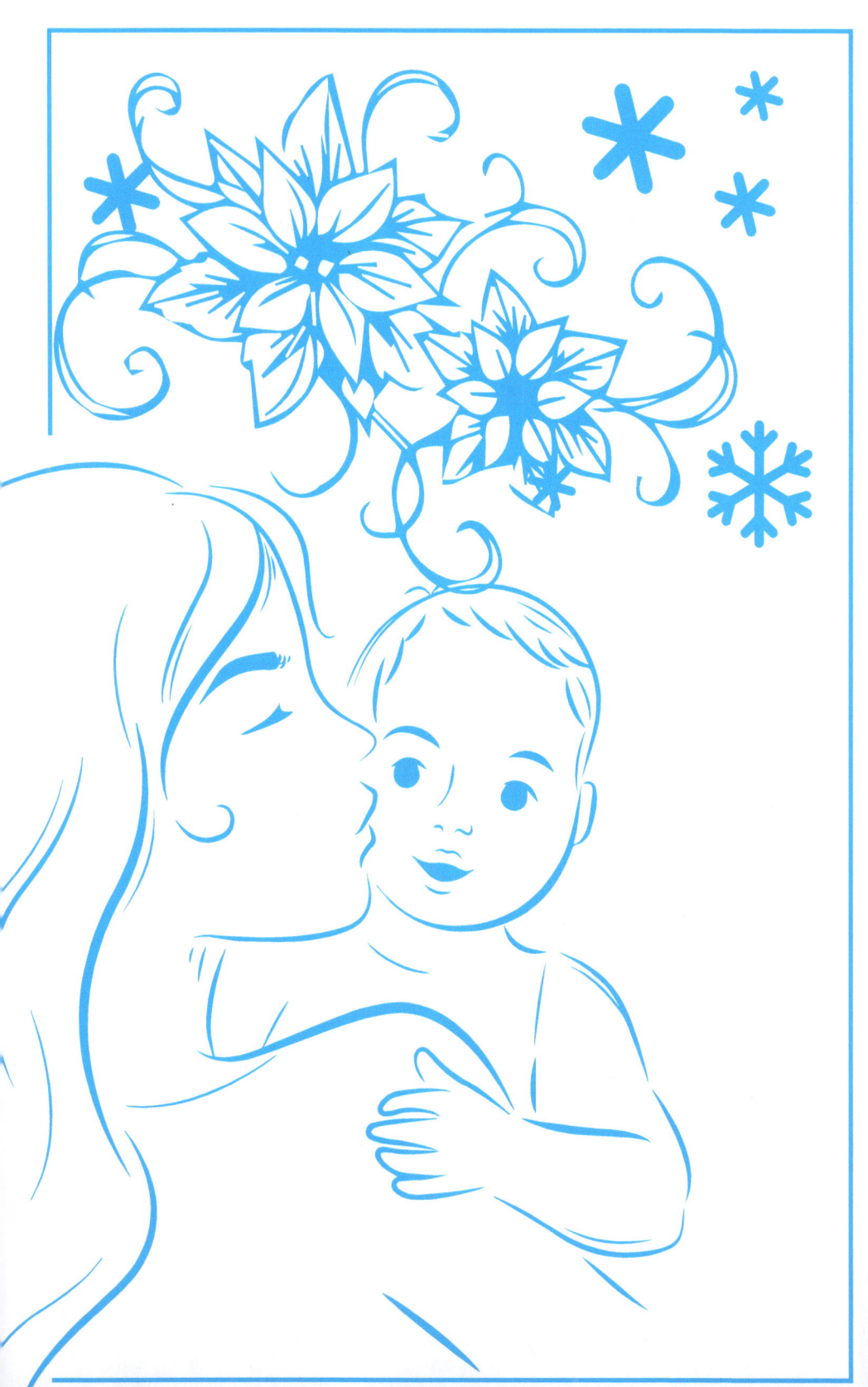

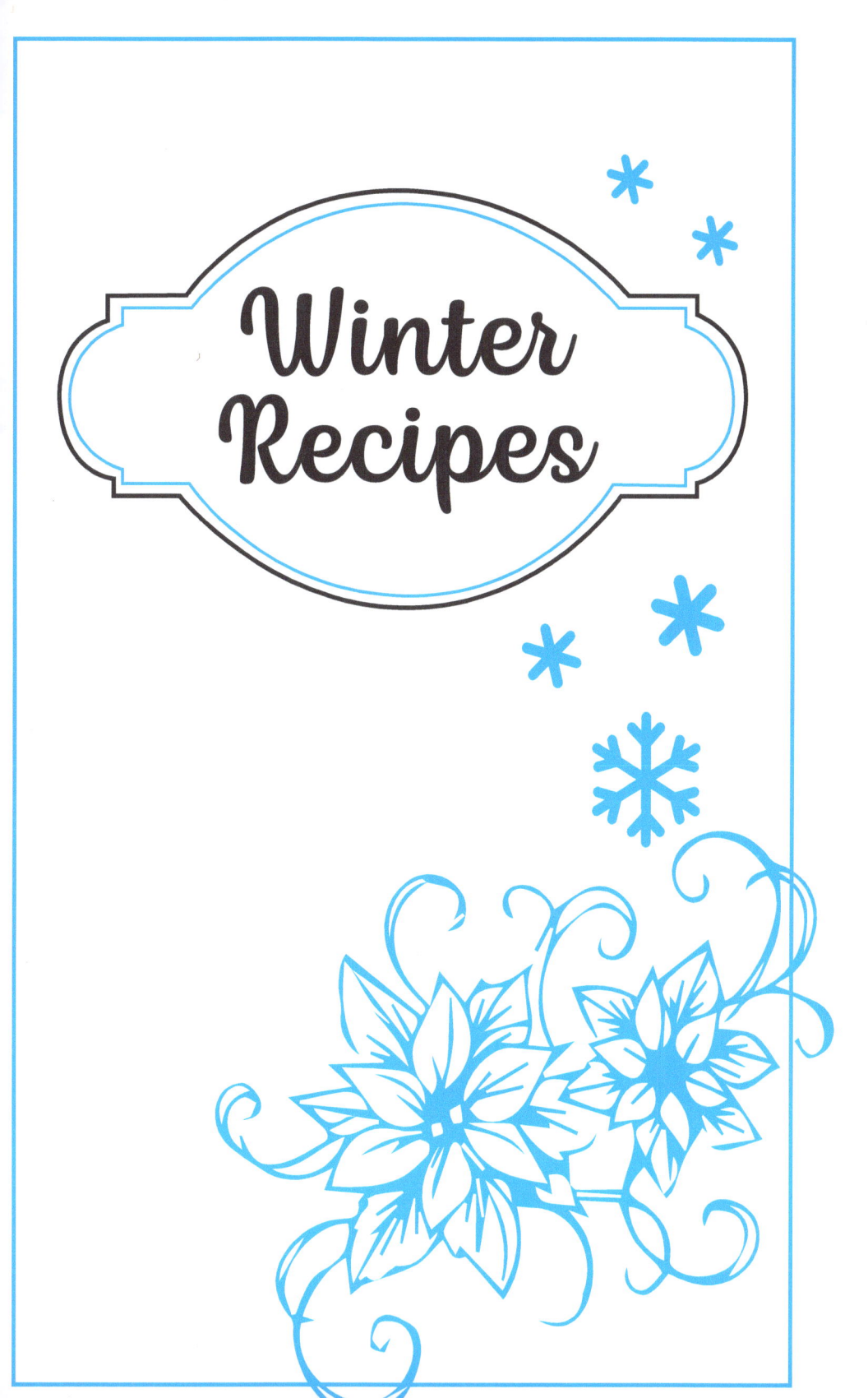

Poached Eggs & Avocado Toast

MAKES 1 SERVING

Ingredients

- 1 Slice Village Bread
- 1 Egg
- 1 Liter Water
- 1 Dessertspoon Apple Cider Vinegar
- Salt
- 1 Tablespoon Condensed Yogurt
- 1 Garlic Clove
- Half Avocado
- Sunflower Seed Kernels
- Black Pepper
- Olive Oil

Directions

1. Boil the water with some salt and apple cider vinegar.
2. Crack the egg carefully into the boiling water, gently poach for 3 minute then lift the egg out of the water with a spatula.
3. Grate the garlic, mix into the yogurt with some salt.
4. Toast the bread and spread with the yogurt mixture, then add the sliced avocado and finally the poached egg on top.
5. Drizzle a little olive oil over the top and sprinkle with sunflower seed kernels. Season with freshly ground black pepper.

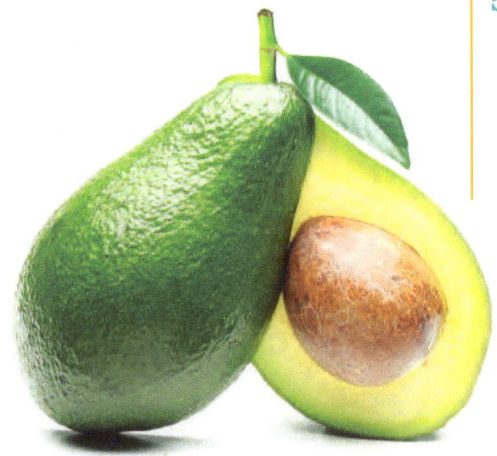

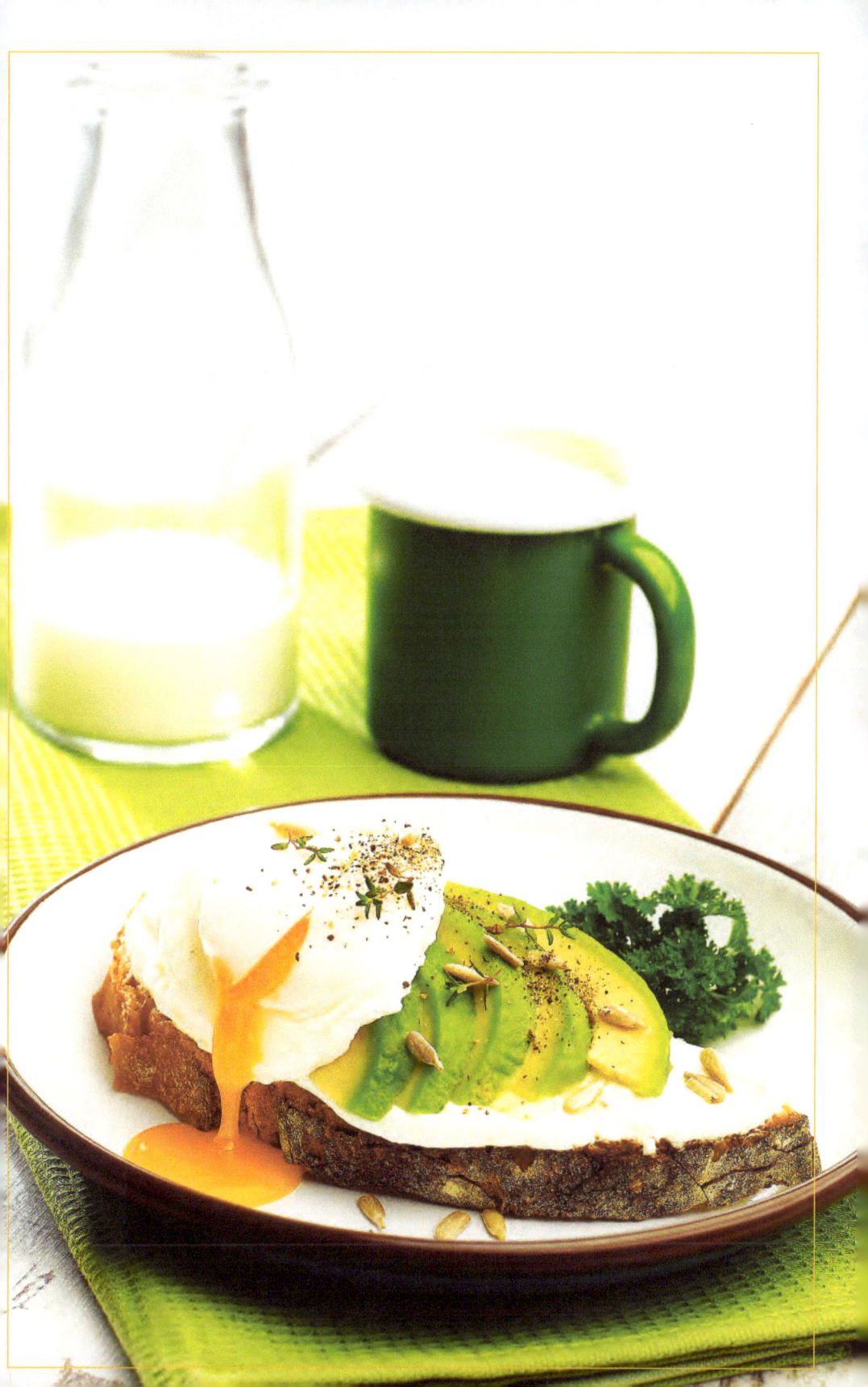

Sunflower Seed Bread

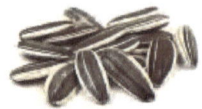

MAKES 6-8 SERVINGS

Ingredients

- 800-900ml Whole Wheat Flour
- 2-3 Dessertspoons Yeast
- 100ml Warm Water
- Salt
- 1 Teaspoon Sugar
- 350ml Warm Water
- 2-3 Tablespoons Sunflower Seed Kernels
- Coconut Oil for the Baking Pan

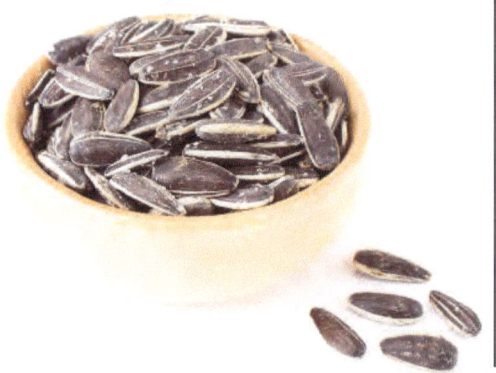

Directions

1. Combine 50ml warm water and the yeast in a bowl, stir a little and let it sit for 10-15 minutes.
2. Place the flour in a deep bowl and pour the water-yeast mixture over it.
3. Mix in the salt, sugar and the warm water, stir an knead until it forms a soft dough.
4. Cover the bowl and allow the dough to rise in a warm place for 40 to 45 minutes.
5. Grease a rectangular baking pan. Preheat oven to 180C.
6. Once the dough has doubled in size, knead it for a short while, then place it in the baking pan. Shape it with your hands, cover the pan and let it rise again for 20 minutes.
7. Sprinkle sunflower seed kernels over the dough, and bake.

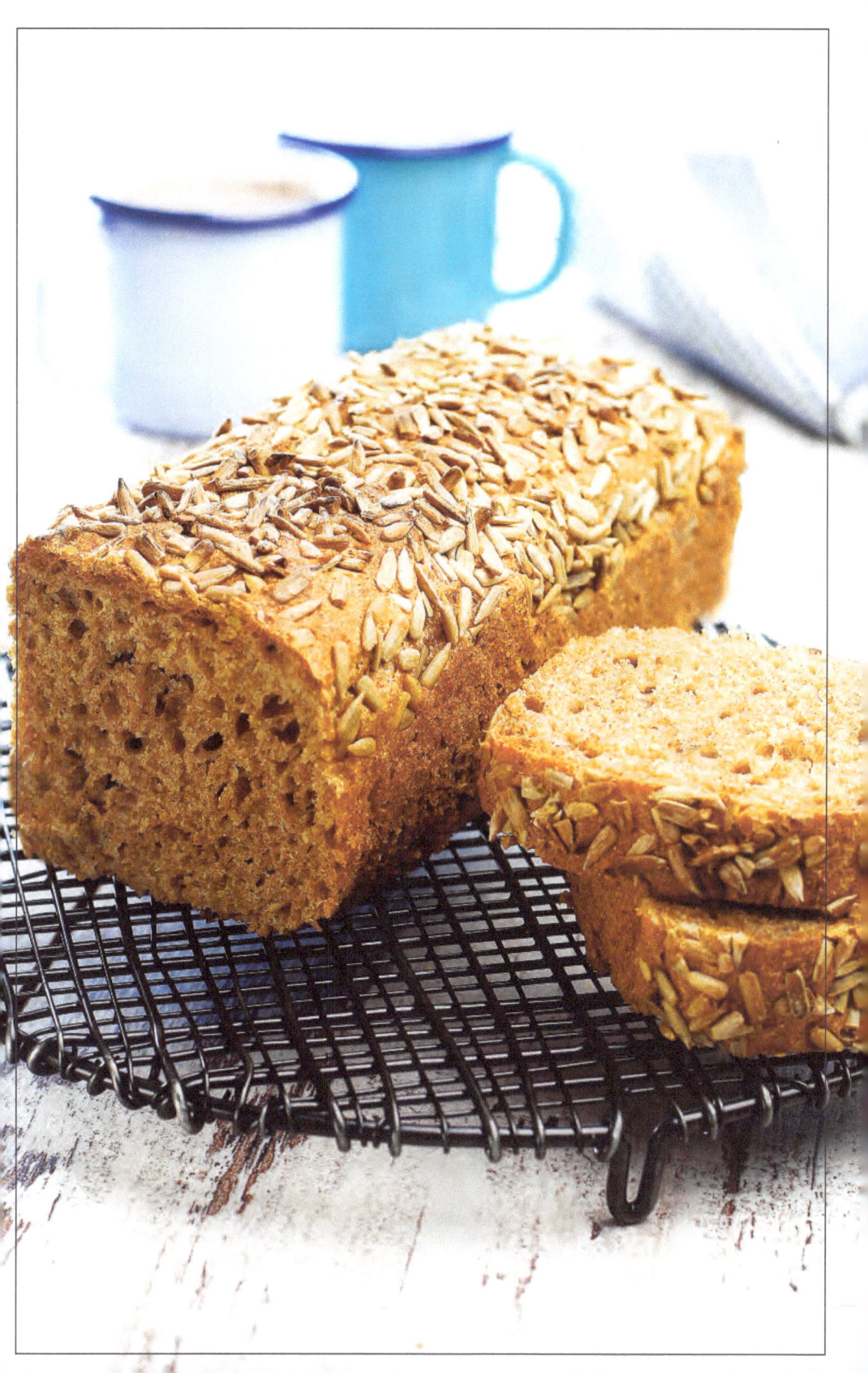

Meat-Stuffed Chard Rolls

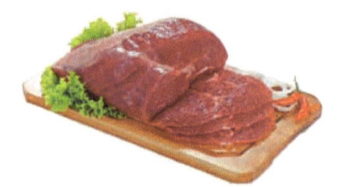

MAKES 6-7 SERVINGS

Ingredients

- 1 Bunch Chard
- 250g Medium Ground Beef
- 90g Siyez (Einkorn) Wheat Bulgur
- 2 Med. Onions, Thinly Chopped
- 1 Tablespoon Tomato Paste
- Salt, Black Pepper
- 1 Teaspoon Cumin
- 5-6 Tablespoons Olive Oil
- 1 Tablespoon Dry Mint
- 2-3 Garlic Cloves
- ½ Bundle Dill, Minced
- ½ Bundle Parsley, Minced
- 200ml Warm Water

For the Sauce
- 600ml Hot Water
- 4 Dessertspoons Tomato Paste
- 80ml Olive Oil

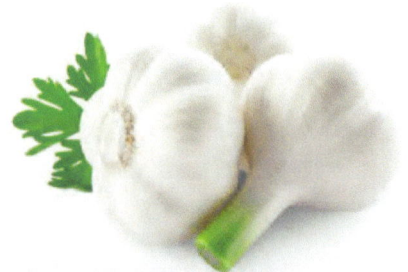

Directions

1. Put the ground beef in a large bowl to prepare the filling.
2. Wash and drain the bulgur, add it to the ground beef.
3. Add the onions. Mix in the tomato paste and red pepper paste, if desired, salt, black pepper, cumin and dry mint.
4. Add olive oil, warm water, and minced garlic. Mix well with a spoon.
4. Add the minced dill and parsley, mix again.
5. In a deep bowl, combine the hot water, tomato paste and olive oil to prepare the sauce.
6. Wash the chard leaves well, cut off the stalks and cover the bottom of your pot with some chard leaves.
7. Put the remaining chard leaves in a large bowl and pour hot water over the leaves.

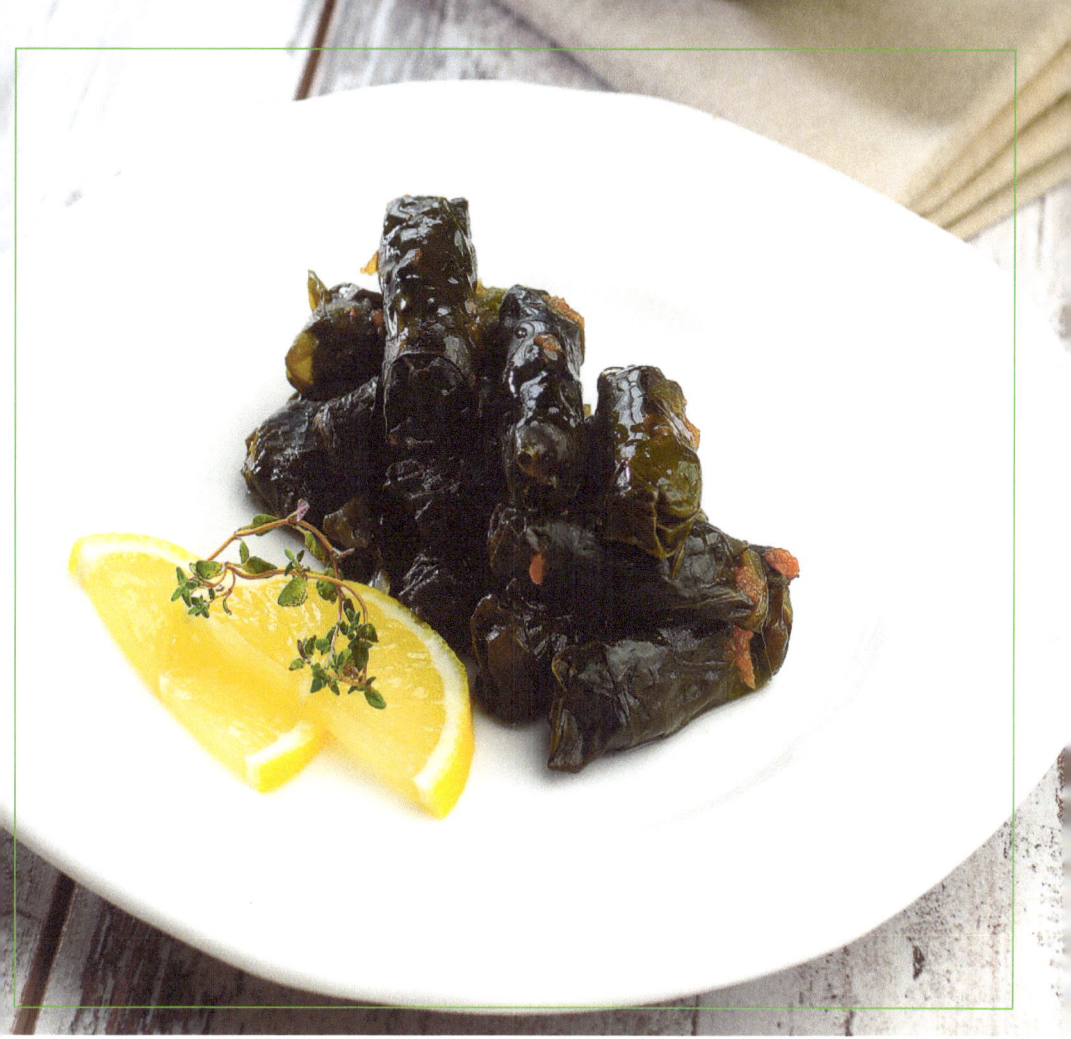

8. Lay the leaves on a flat surface, bright side down.
9. Place one tablespoon of ground beef stuffing on the large side of each leaf, fold in the sides and then roll into a log. Do the same for the rest of the chard leaves.
9. In the pot, arrange the rolls side by side in layers.
10. Pour the tomato paste sauce over the rolls and weigh the rolls down with a porcelain plate.
11. Cook over medium heat until the liquid comes to a boil.
12. Turn the heat to low and cook for 20-25 minutes until rolls are tender.
13. Serve hot.
14. If desired, pour garlic yogurt over the rolls.

Hummus

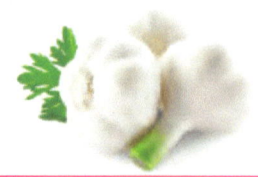

MAKES 4-5 SERVINGS

Ingredients

- 200ml Chickpeas
- 4 Tablespoons Tahini
- 1 Lemon
- 3-4 Garlic Cloves
- 2 Tablespoons Olive Oil
- 2 Tablespoons Water
- Sea Salt
- Cumin

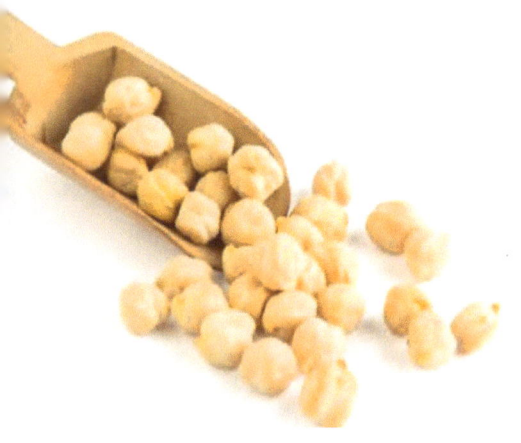

Directions

1. Wash the chickpeas and soak them in water overnight.
2. Drain the chickpeas, cover them with water and boil.
3. Repeat the process again, this time boil until chickpeas are soft.
4. Peel off the skins of the chickpeas.
5. Mix tahini, lemon juice, olive oil, garlic, salt and cumin in a food processor.
6. Add in half of the chickpeas and mix until creamy.
7. Add the rest of the chickpeas and process it all.
8. Transfer to a serving plate.
9. Drizzle olive oil over.
10. Ready to serve!

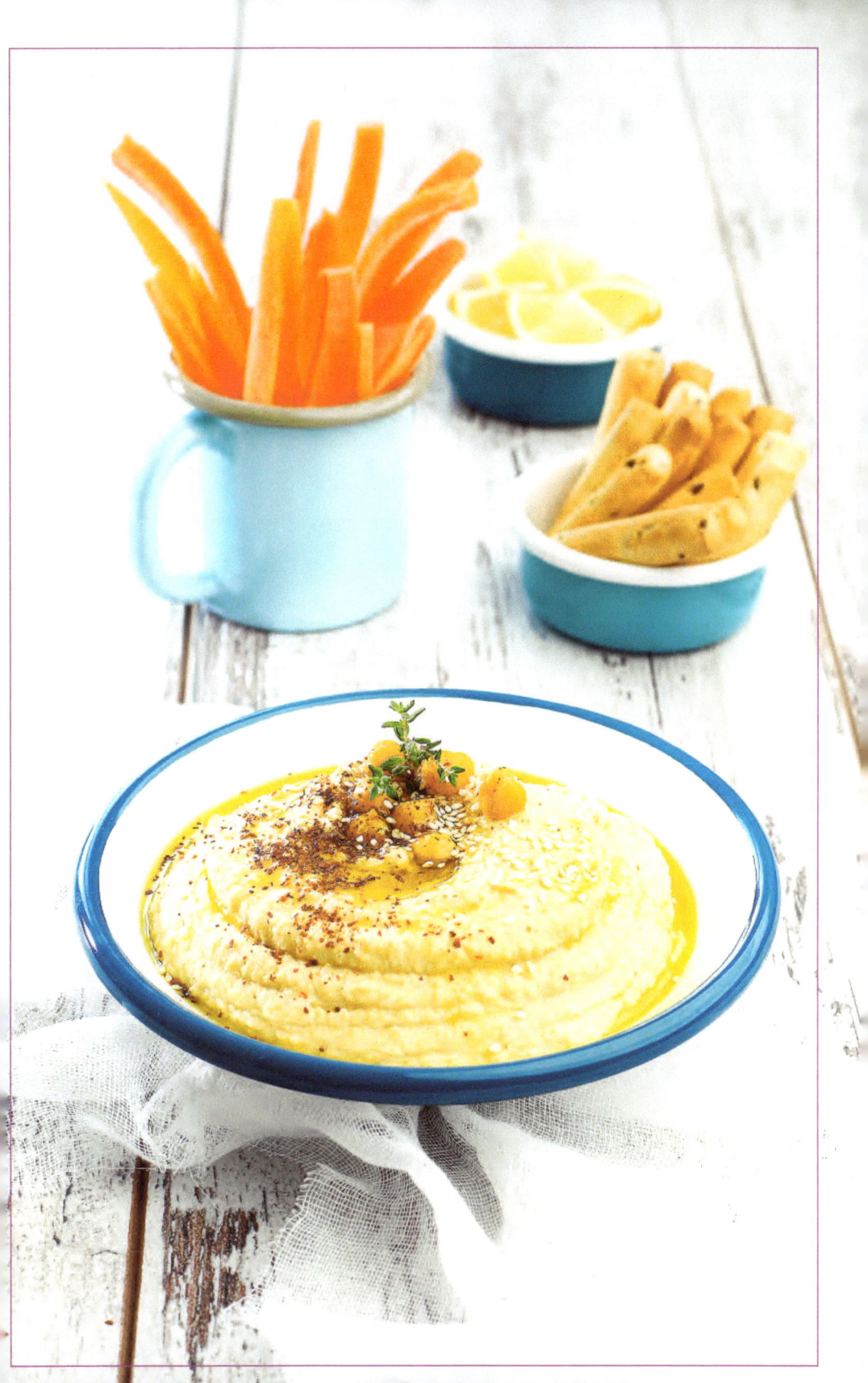

Salmon with Dates

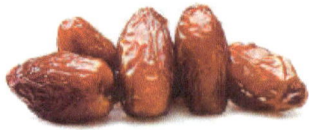

MAKES 2 SERVINGS

Ingredients

- 2 Salmon Fillets
- 6 Dates
- 2 Tablespoons Raw Almonds
- 2 Tablespoons Coconut Oil
- Salt
- Black Pepper

Directions

1. Finely chop the pitted dates and almonds.
2. Place the salmon fillets on a sheet of parchment paper.
3. Drizzle a spoon of coconut oil over each fillet.
4. Season with salt and pepper.
5. Sprinkle the date-almond mixture evenly over the fillets.
6. Cover the baking pan with the parchment paper.
7. Bake in the oven at 200C for 30 minutes.

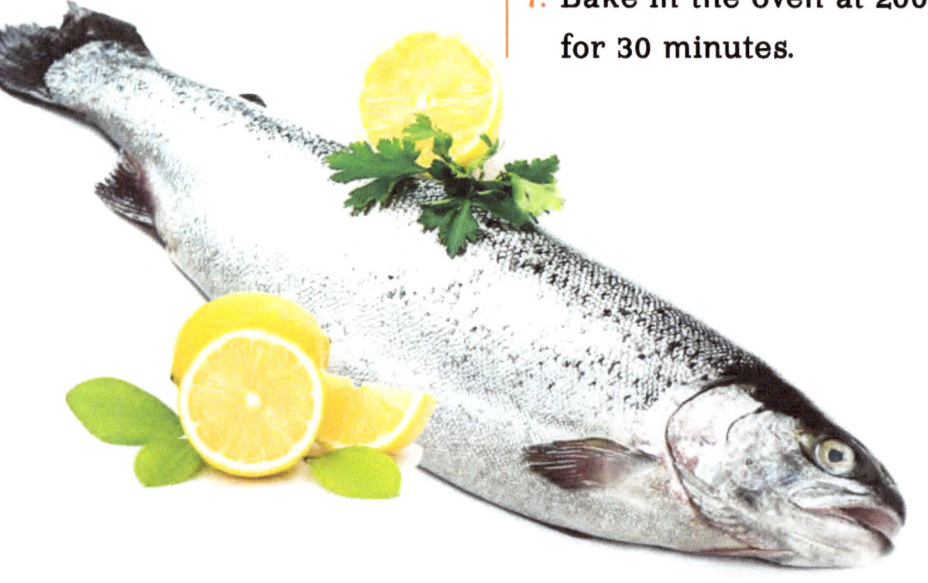

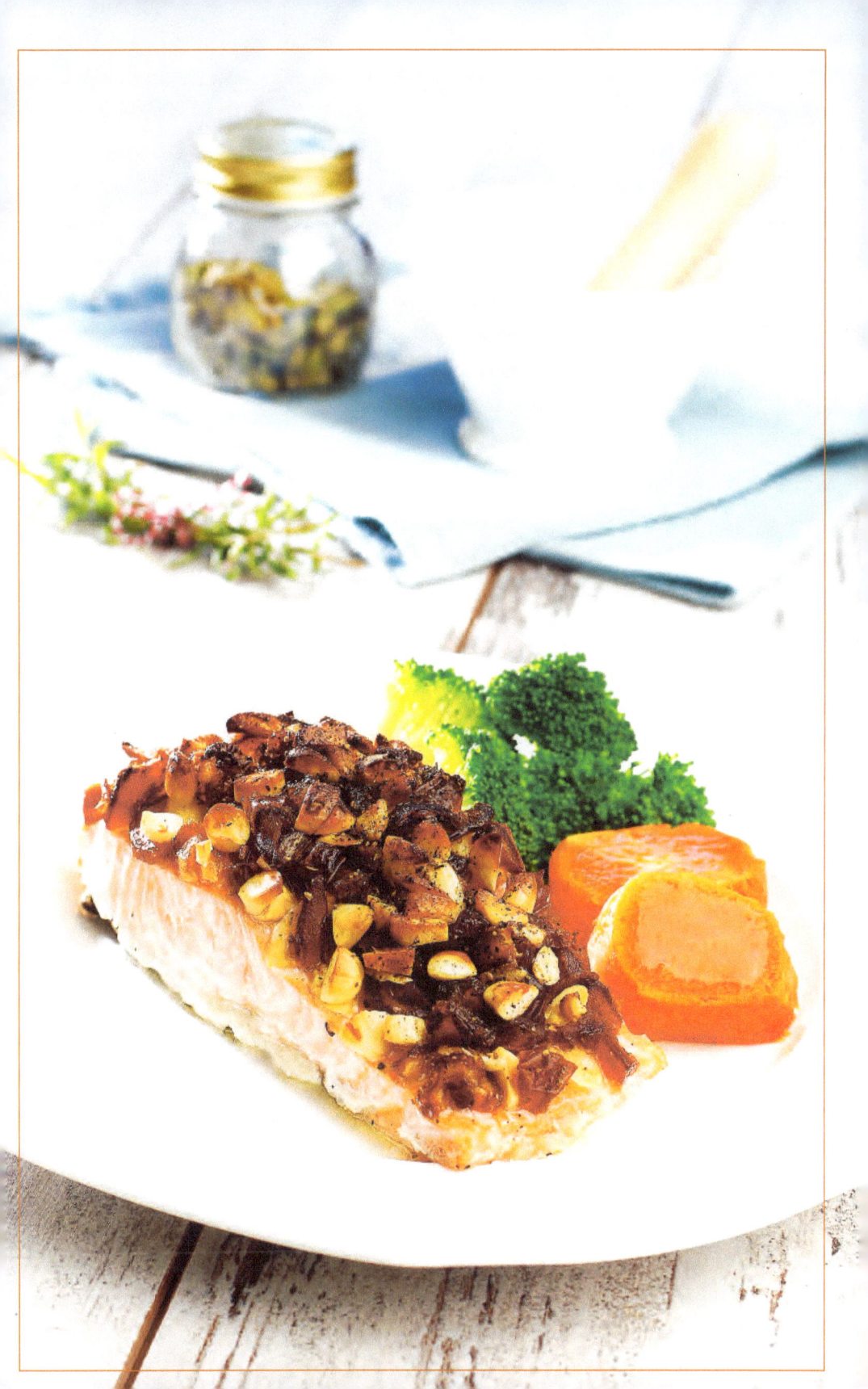

Zucchini Soup in Lemon Egg Sauce

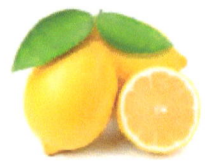

MAKES 4 SERVINGS

Ingredients

- 3 Zucchini
- 1 Large Onion
- 1 1/2 Liters Water
- 2 Tablespoons Coconut Oil
- 2-3 Garlic Cloves
- Salt
- Whole Black Pepper
- Dill

For the Sauce

- 1 Egg
- 1/2 Lemon, Juiced

Directions

1. Prepare the zucchini, garlic, and onion, cut into large pieces and put in a pot.
2. Add the remaining main ingredients except the dill and cook until the vegetables are completely soft.
3. Blend well in a blender.
4. Transfer the mixture back into the pot.
5. Whisk the egg and the lemon juice well in a bowl.
6. Add several spoonfuls of the hot soup into the mixture to warm it.
7. Slowly add the mixture to the soup. Stir and bring to a boil.
8. Sprinkle the minced dill over the soup and serve.

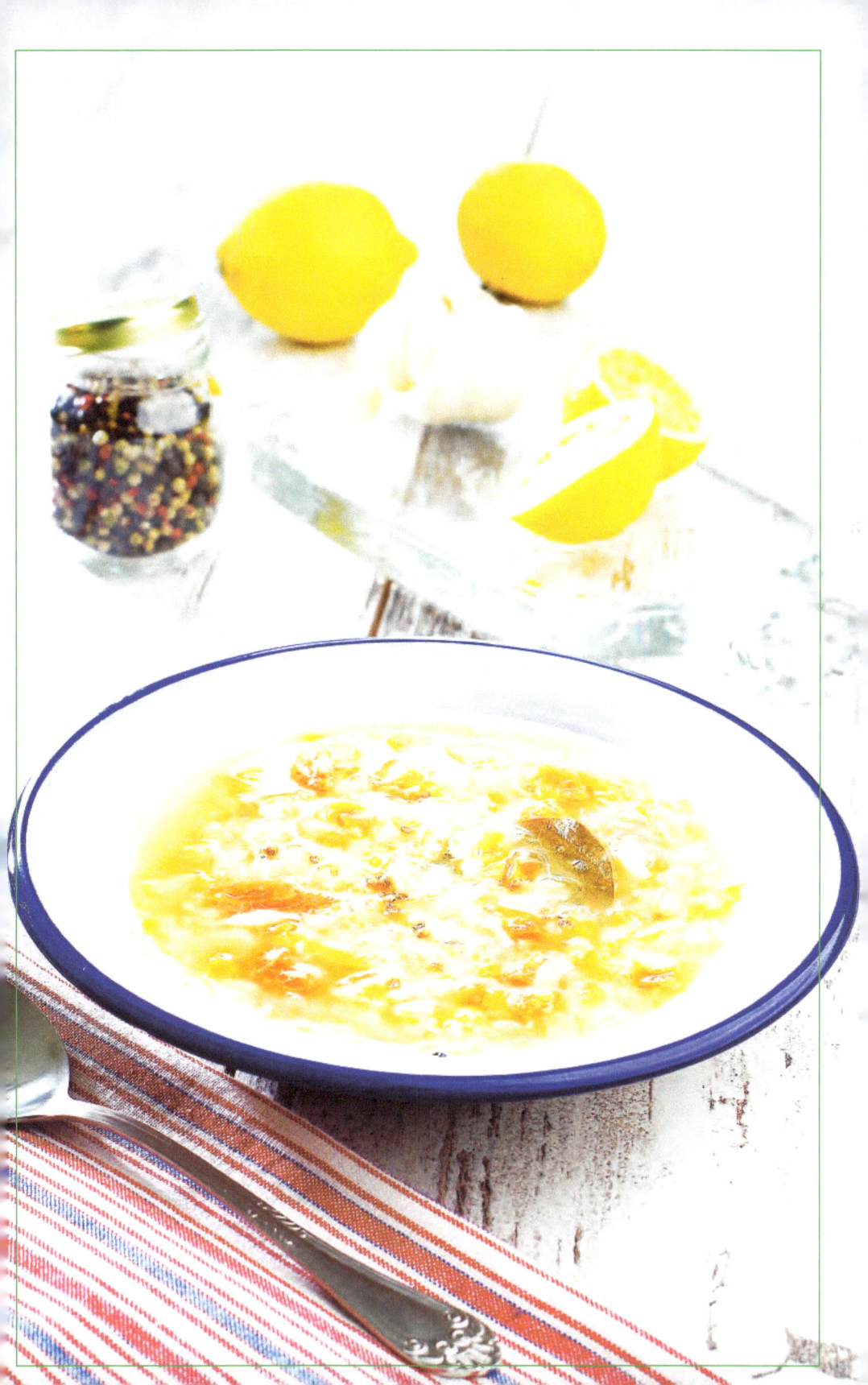

Apricot Slices

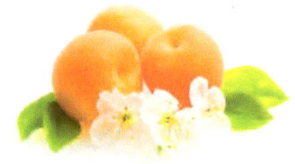

MAKES 6-8 SERVINGS

Ingredients

- 150g Dried Apricots
- 10-12 Cardamom Pods (release seeds by cracking open pods)
- 5 Dates
- 100g Cashews
- 200g Almond-Walnut-Hazelnut Mixture
- 3 Tablespoons Shredded Coconut

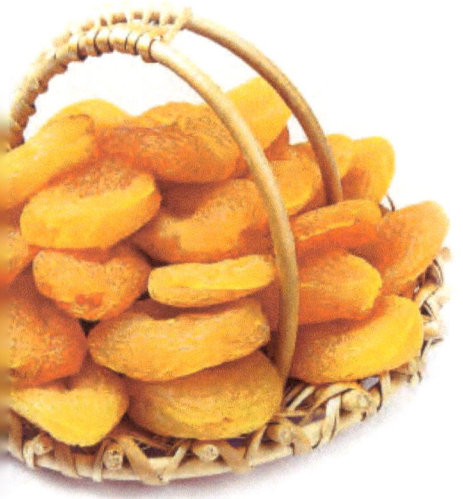

Directions

1. Combine the cashews with half of the almond-walnut-hazelnut mixture in a food processor and process for 30 seconds.
2. Add apricots, pitted dates cardamom seeds, and shredded coconut, and grind for another 2 minutes
3. When the mixture becomes consistent like a dough, place it between two pieces of parchment paper and roll out to your desired thickness.
4. Chop the rest of the almond-walnut-hazelnut mixture in the processor and sprinkle over the dough.
5. Slice into pieces of desired size before placing in the refrigerator. Chill for 2 hours before serving.
6. Slices can also be stored in an airtight container in the refrigerator.

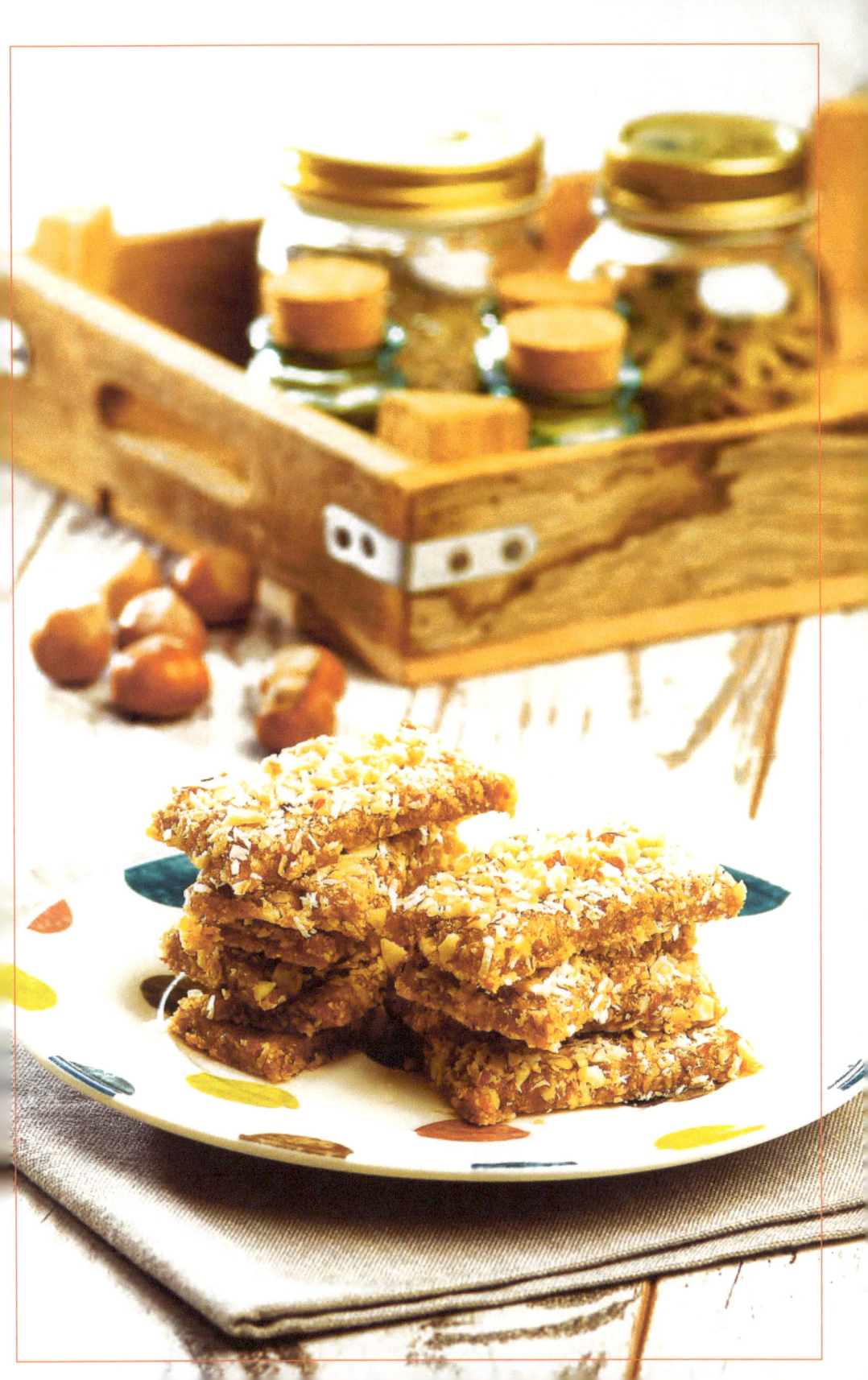

Winter Vegetable Soup with Beef Broth

MAKES 5-6 SERVINGS

Ingredients

- 1 Tablespoon Coconut Oil
- 1 Onion
- 1 Leek
- 1 Carrot, Diced
- 8 Broccoli Florets
- 1½ Liters Water
- 1 Small Bowl Beef Broth
- 1 Tablespoon Brown Rice
- 3 Tablespoons Boiled Chickpeas
- Salt
- Cumin
- Whole Black Peppercorns

Directions

1. Melt the coconut oil in a pot.
2. Add the chopped onion into the pot, stirring continually. Cook for several minutes.
3. Add thinly sliced leek and continue cooking.
4. Add the water, beef broth, diced carrots, broccoli florets, whole black peppercorns, brown rice, and boiled chickpeas to the pot.
5. Season with salt and cumin when vegetables are soft.
6. Serve hot.

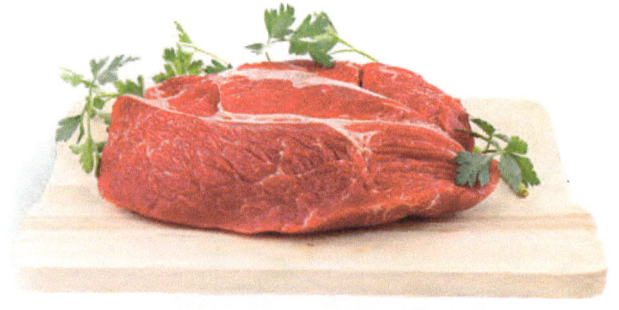

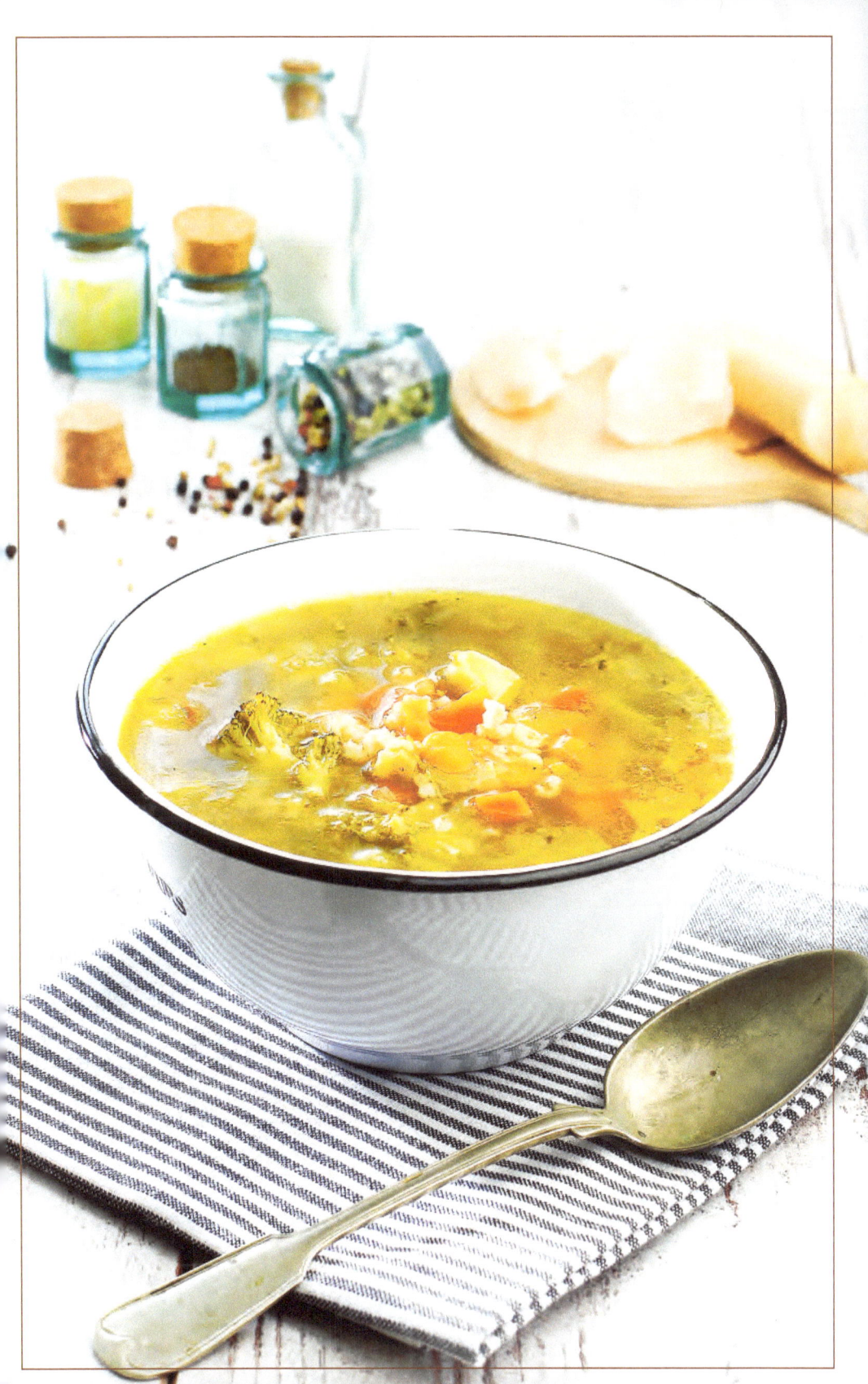

Winter Salad

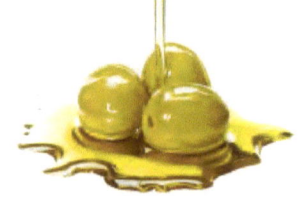

MAKES 3-4 SERVINGS

Ingredients

- ½ Bunch Spinach
- 1 Turnip Radish
- Orange
- Sunflower Seeds
- Goat Cheese
- Olive Oil
- Lemon
- Salt

Directions

1. Grate the turnip radish, thinly slice the spinach, slice the orange.
2. Combine all ingredients season with olive oil, lemon, and salt.
3. Toss to coat.

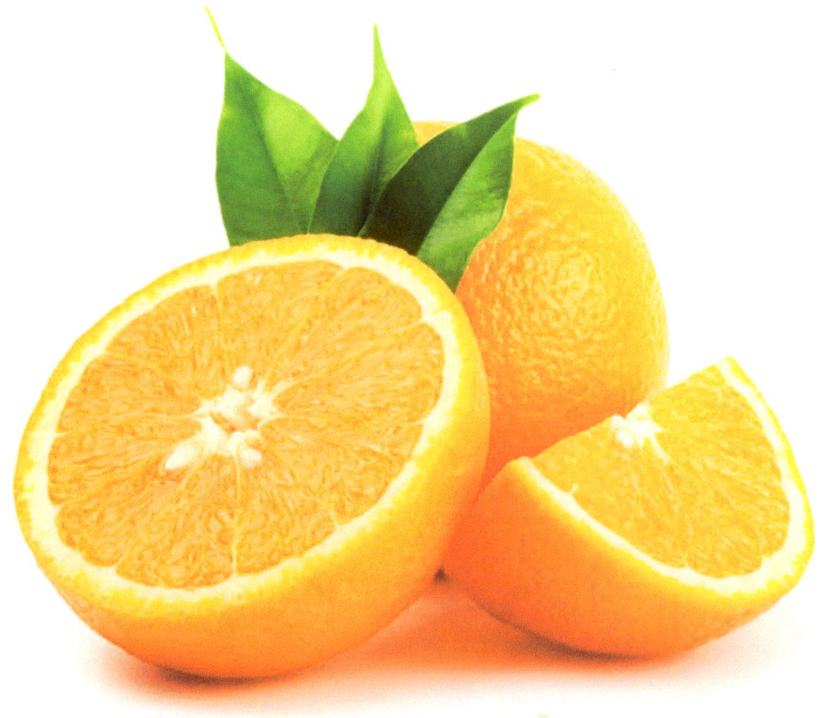

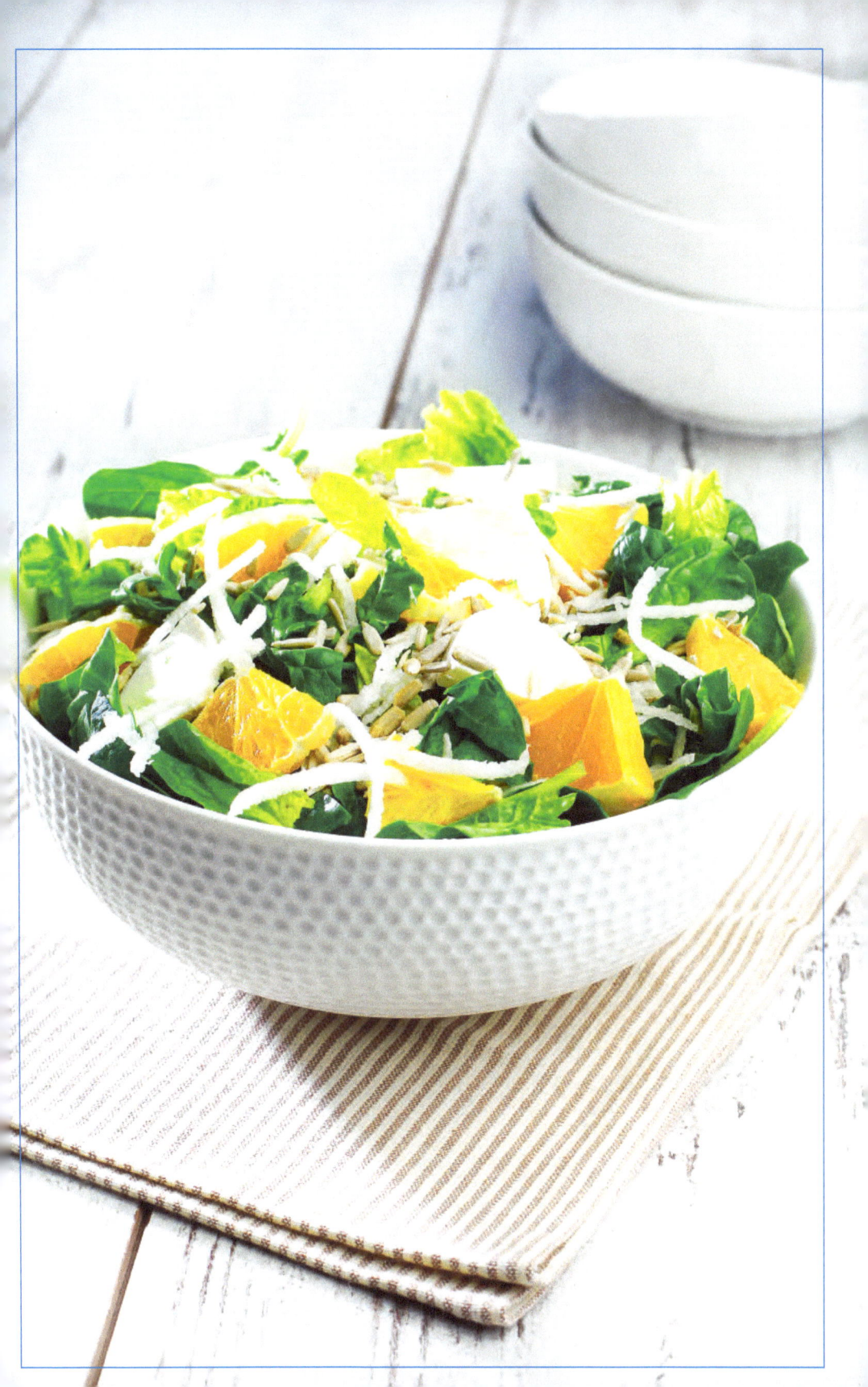

Masala Chai

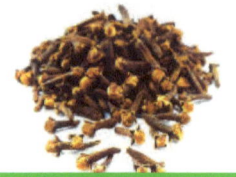

MAKES 2 SERVINGS

Ingredients

- 5-6 Cardamom Pods
- 2-3 Clove Buds
- 1 Stick Cinnamon
- 6-7 Whole Black Peppercorns
- 1 Whole Star Anise
- ½ Teaspoon Grated Nutmeg
- 180ml Milk
- 240ml Water
- ½ Teaspoon Masala Powder (optional)
- 1 Coffee Spoon Black Tea
- A Bit of Fresh Ginger

Directions

1. Put the herbs in a teapot and boil for a couple of minutes.
2. Add the ginger, masala and the black tea and boil 2-3 minutes.
4. Add the milk and boil an extra 2-3 minutes.
5. Use a tea strainer to serve.

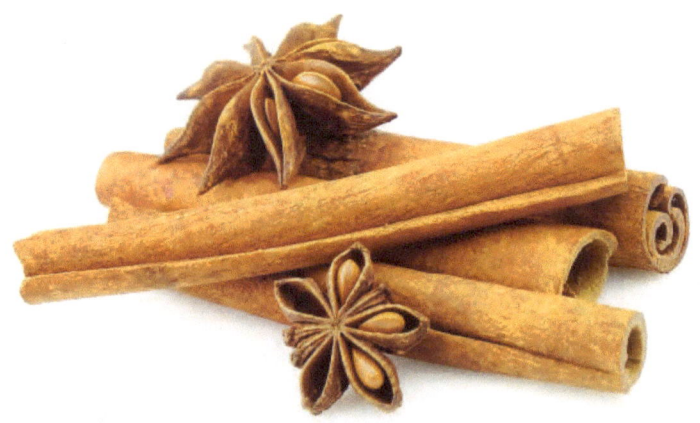

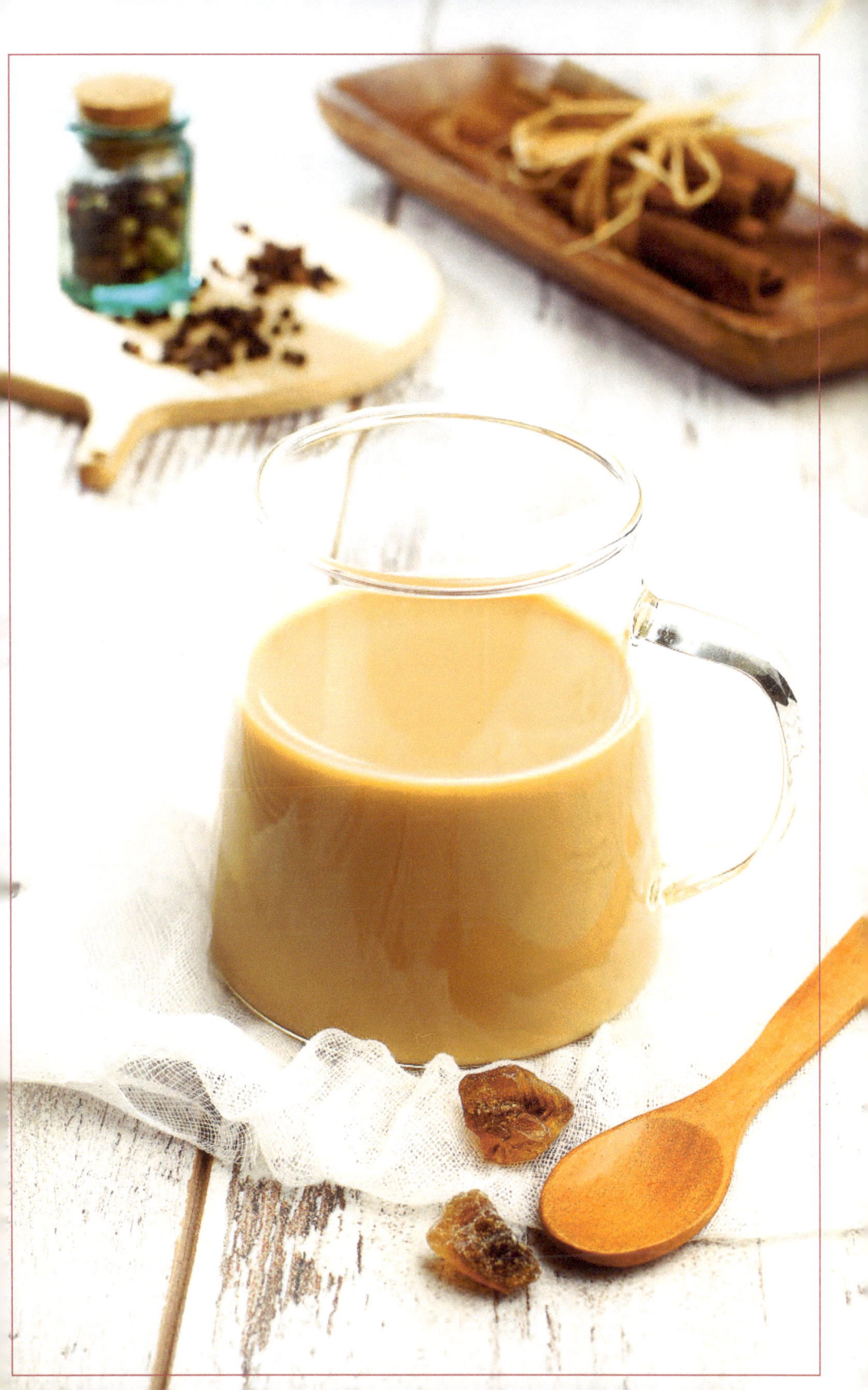

Sugar-Free Pumpkin Dessert

MAKES 4 SERVINGS

Ingredients

- 2 Slices Pumpkin
- Small Amount of Water
- Clotted Cream (Turkish Cream)
- Walnuts

Directions

1. Preheat the oven to 180C.
2. Add a small amount of water at the bottom of a baking pan.
3. Place the pumpkin slices in the pan and bake in the preheated oven until tender.
4. Allow the pumpkin slices to cool.
5. Serve with coarsely chopped walnuts and clotted cream.

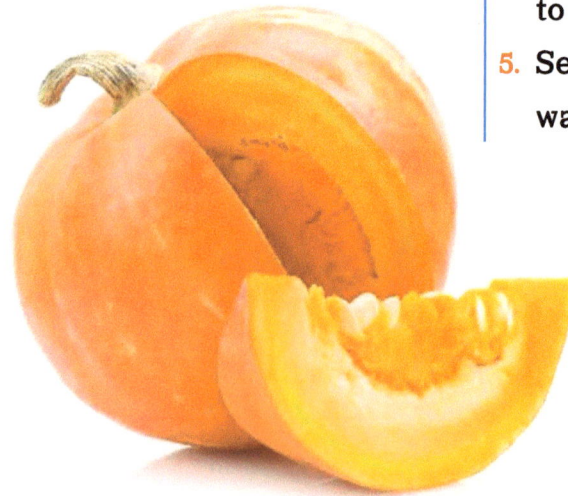

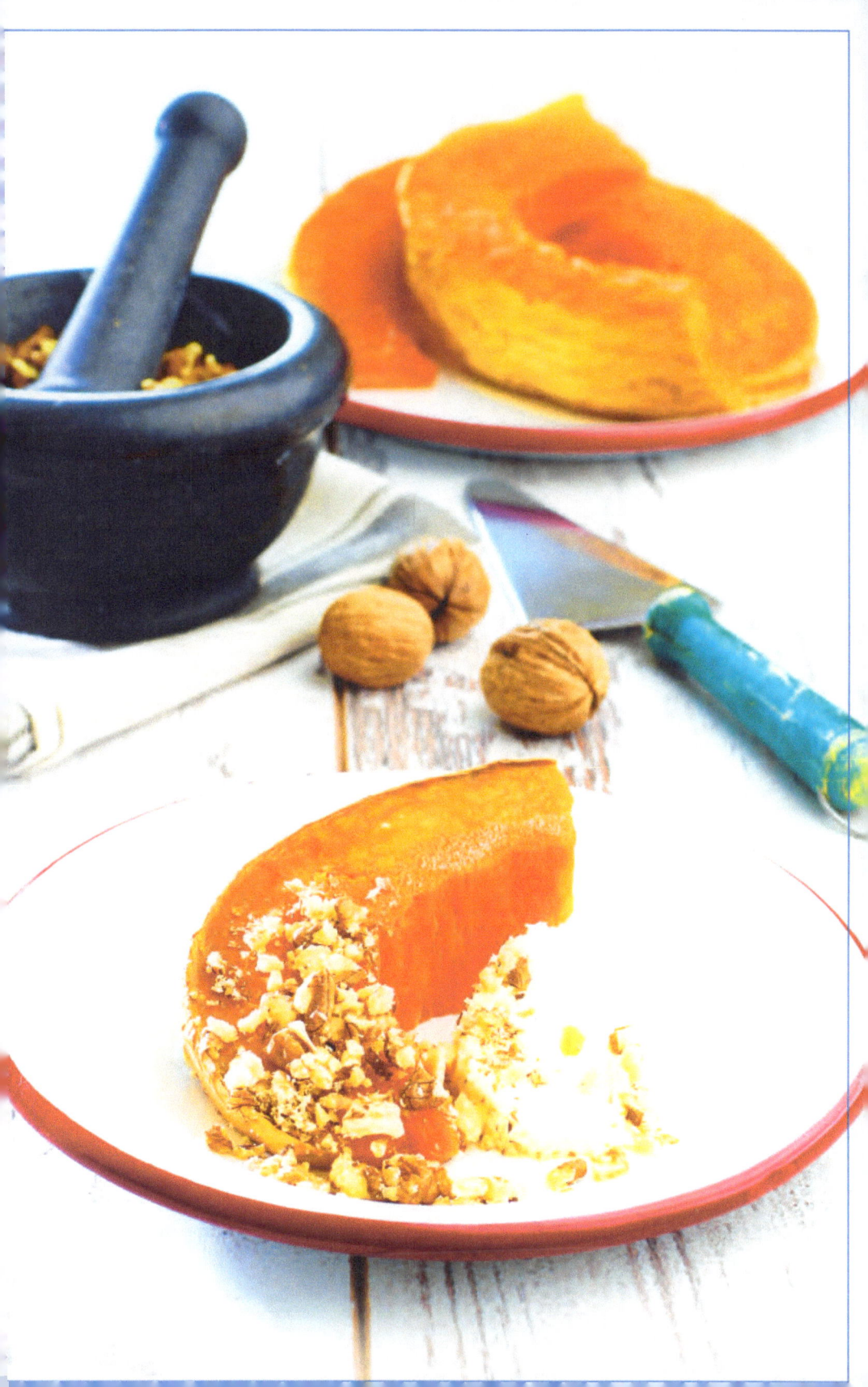

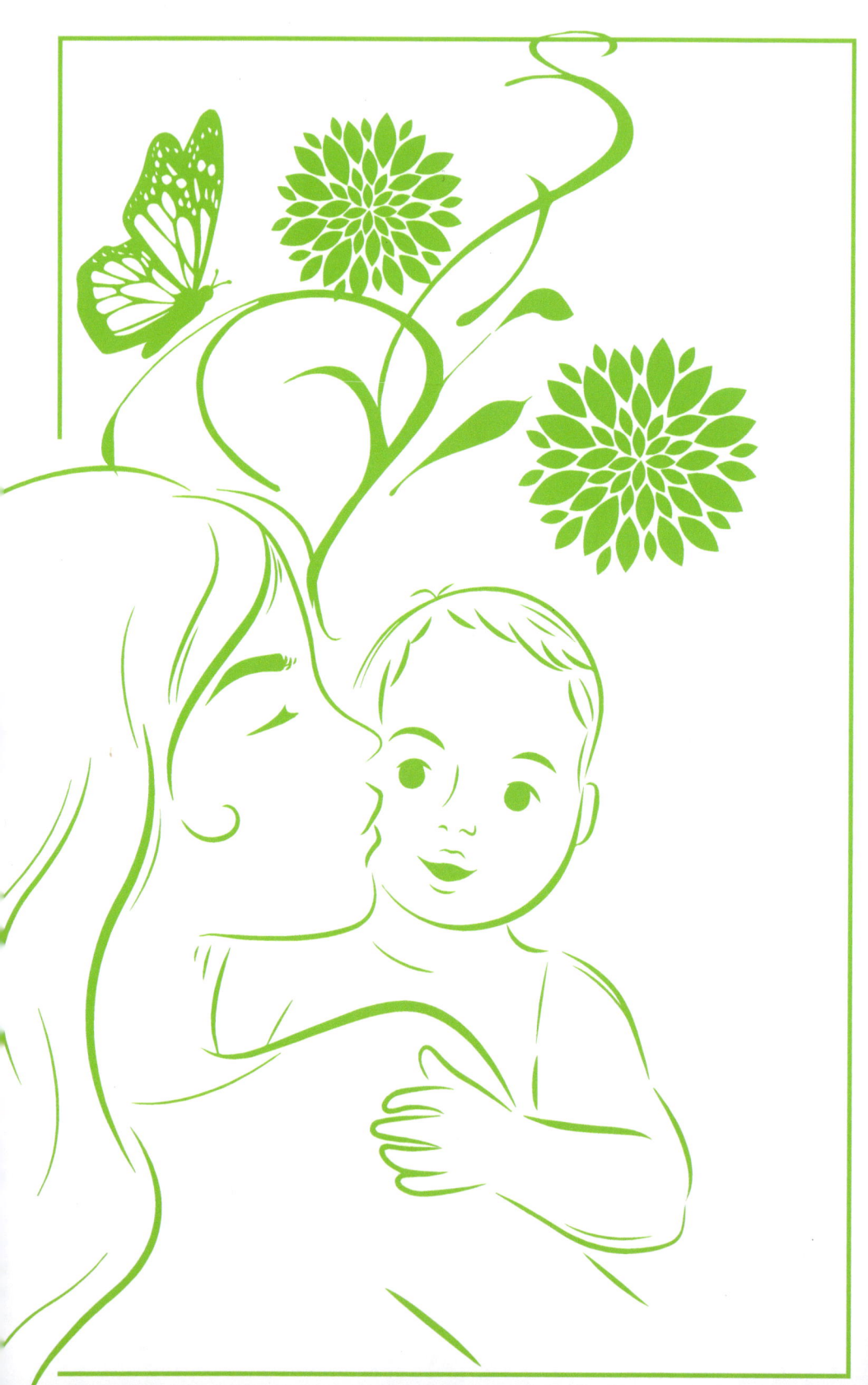

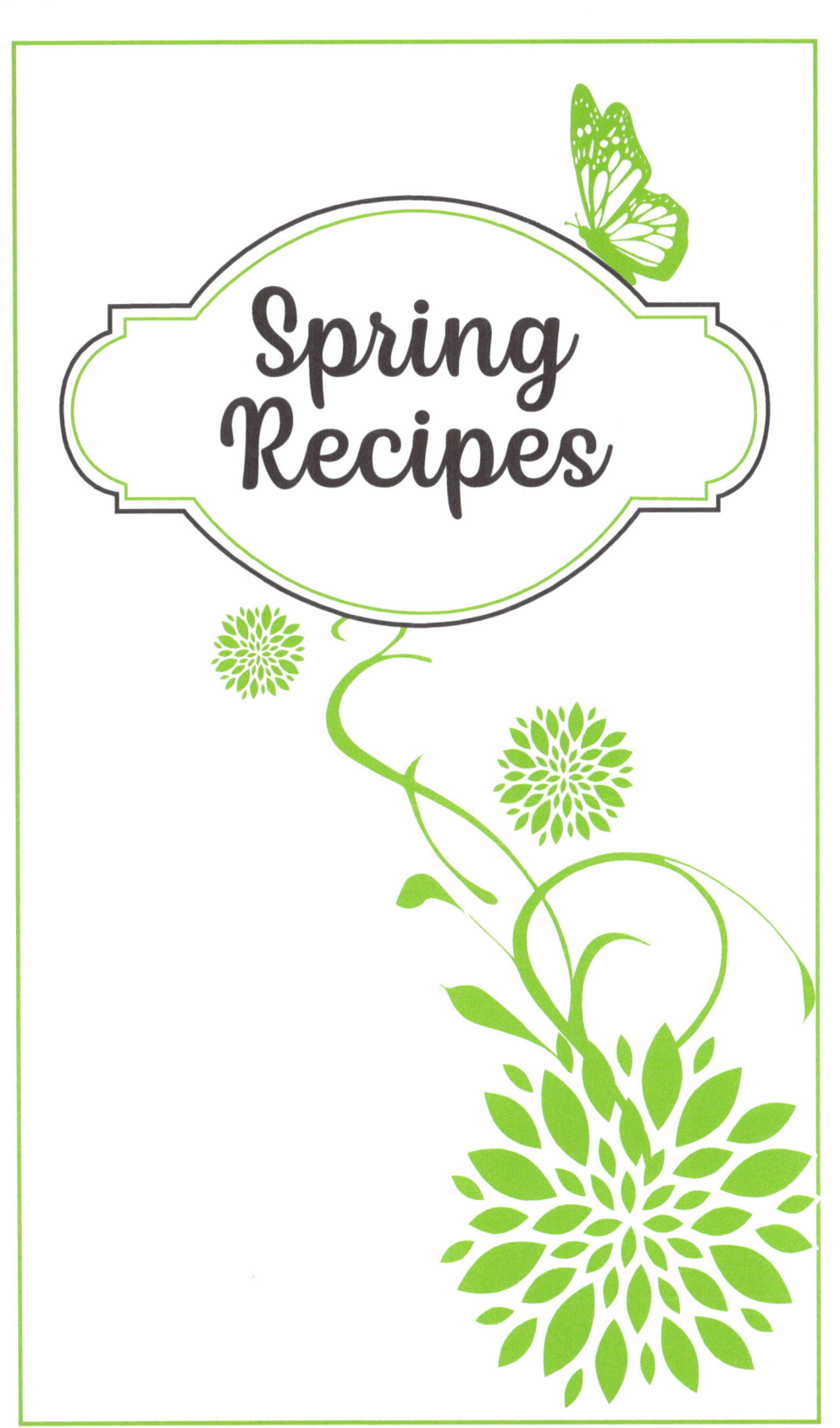

Fish Soup

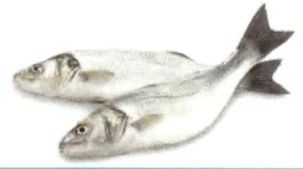

MAKES 4-5 SERVINGS

Ingredients

- 1 Sea Bass
- 1 ½ Liter Water
- 2 Onions
- 1 Carrot
- 1 Leek
- 3-4 Garlic Cloves
- 1 Celery Root
- Sea Salt
- Whole Black Pepper
- Coriander Seeds
- 2-3 Bay Leaves
- Olive Oil
- Lemon Juice

Directions

1. Combine the cleaned, washed and cut-up fish, 1 onion, bay leaves, whole black peppers and water in a pot.
2. Boil until fish is cooked, then, with a spatula, separate the meat from the bones, set aside.
3. Put the head and fish bones back into the pot and boil for another 30 minutes.
4. Clean the remaining onion, carrot, leek and garlic cloves and dice.
5. Pick the fish meat to shreds.
6. Strain the fish broth, discarding head and bones.
7. Transfer the diced ingredients and the strained fish broth back into the pot and cook until the vegetables are tender.
8. Just before removing from heat, add a little olive oil and season with salt to taste.
9. Serve with lemon juice and freshly ground black pepper.

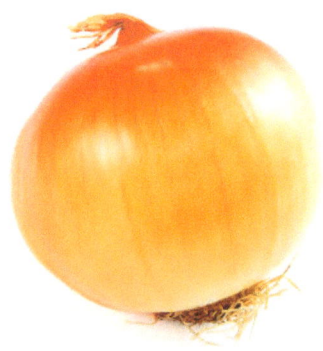

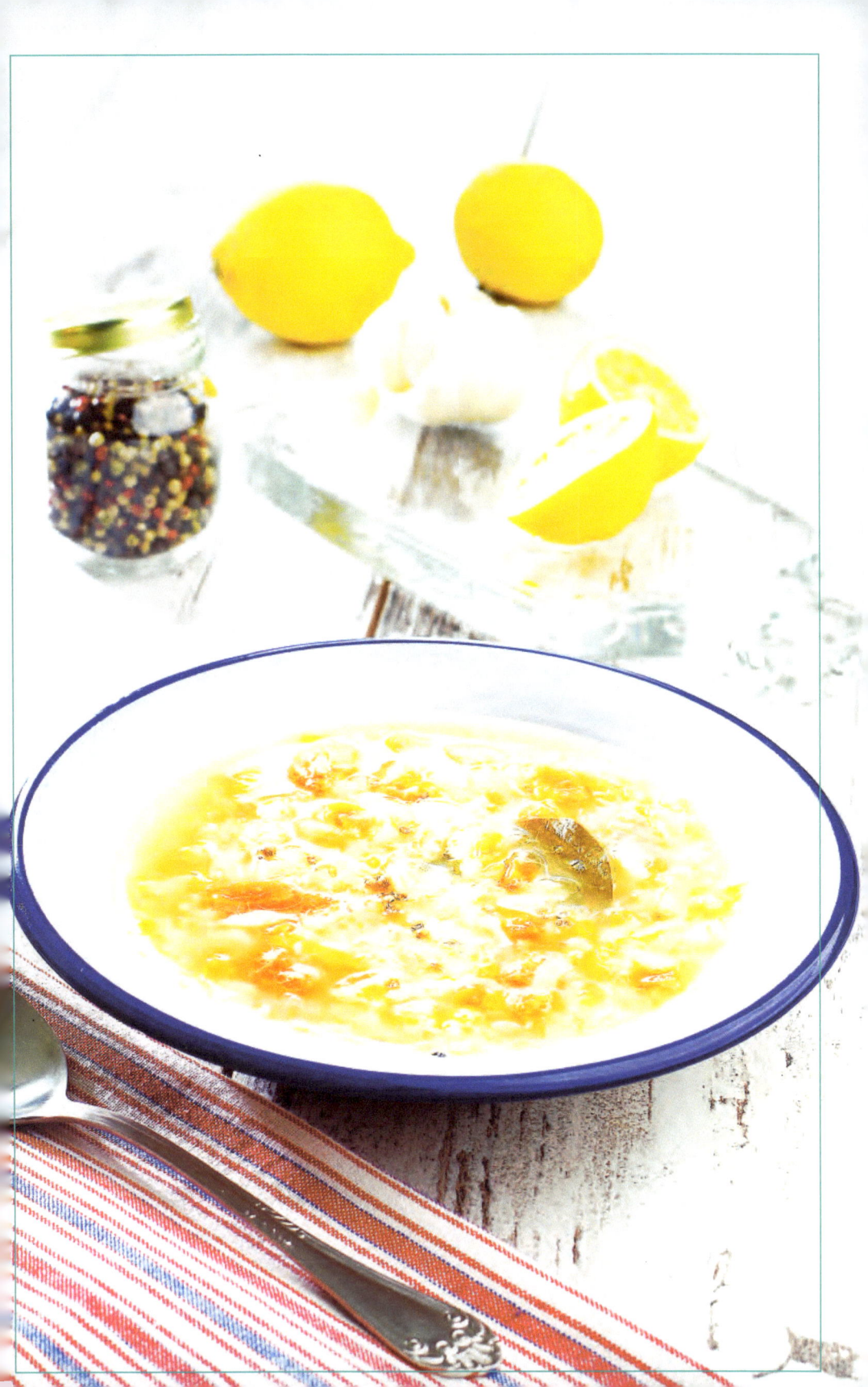

English Pea Salad with Goat Cheese

MAKES 6 SERVINGS

Ingredients

- 1 kg Fresh Peas
- 1/4 Bundle Dill
- Olive Oil
- 1 Tablespoon Lemon Juice
- Salt
- 3-4 Slices Goat Cheese

Directions

1. Crack open the pea pods to free the peas.
2. Transfer them to a colander, then place it on a pot filled with boiling water and cover, steaming the peas until slightly tender.
3. Combine peas with minced dill, olive oil, lemon juice and salt in a separate bowl.
4. Serve with goat cheese crumbled over the top.

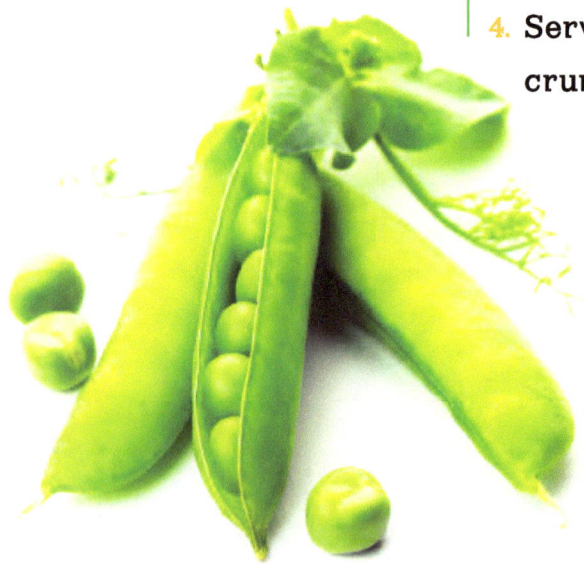

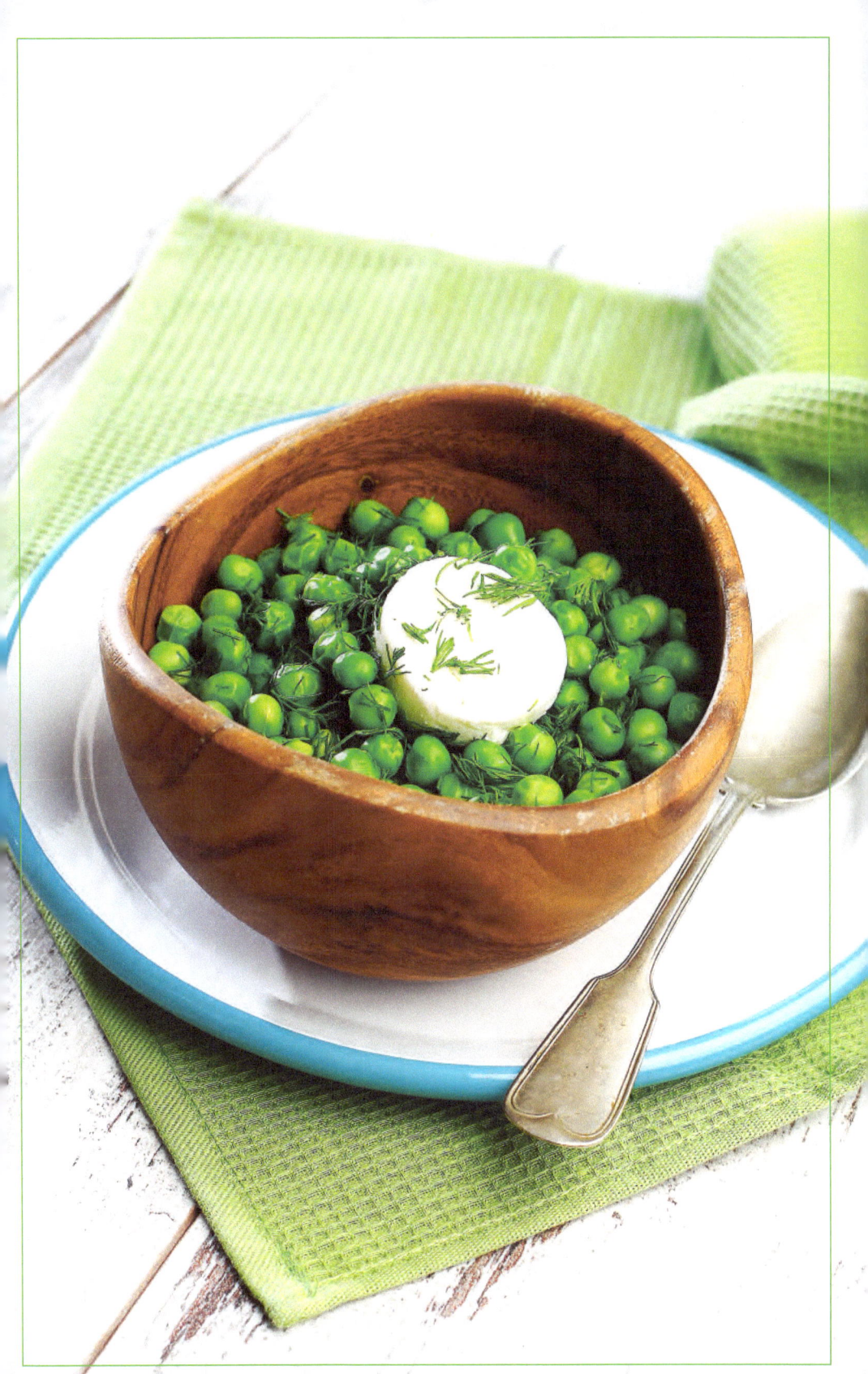

Granola

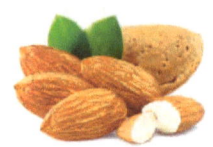

MAKES 6-7 SERVINGS

Ingredients

- 400ml Oats
- 200ml Raw Almonds
- 100ml Sunflower Seed Kernels
- 2-3 Tablespoons Sesame
- 2-3 Tablespoons Flax Seed
- 3 Teaspoons Cinnamon
- 1 Pinch Salt
- 1 Apple, Peeled, Cored and Chopped
- 4 Tablespoons Grape Molasses
- 2 Tablespoons Honey
- 1 Tablespoon Olive Oil
- 100ml Dried Cranberries or Raisins

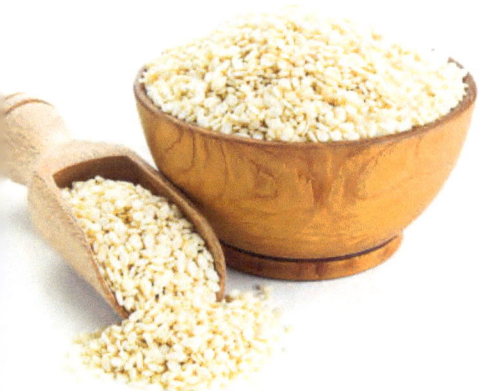

Directions

1. Combine all the dry ingredients in a bowl.
2. Puree the apple and mix with molasses, honey and olive oil, then add the mixture to the dry ingredients.
3. Preheat the oven to 150C.
4. Cover a baking tray with parchment paper, spread the mixture in a thin layer on the paper and bake in the oven for 40 minutes, tossing occasionally.
5. Add cranberries or raisins, if desired, after taking the mixture out of the oven.
6. Granola can be stored in an airtight container or mason jar for a long time.
7. You can double or triple the measure for a larger amount but make sure not to bake it all in one tray or it will stick together.

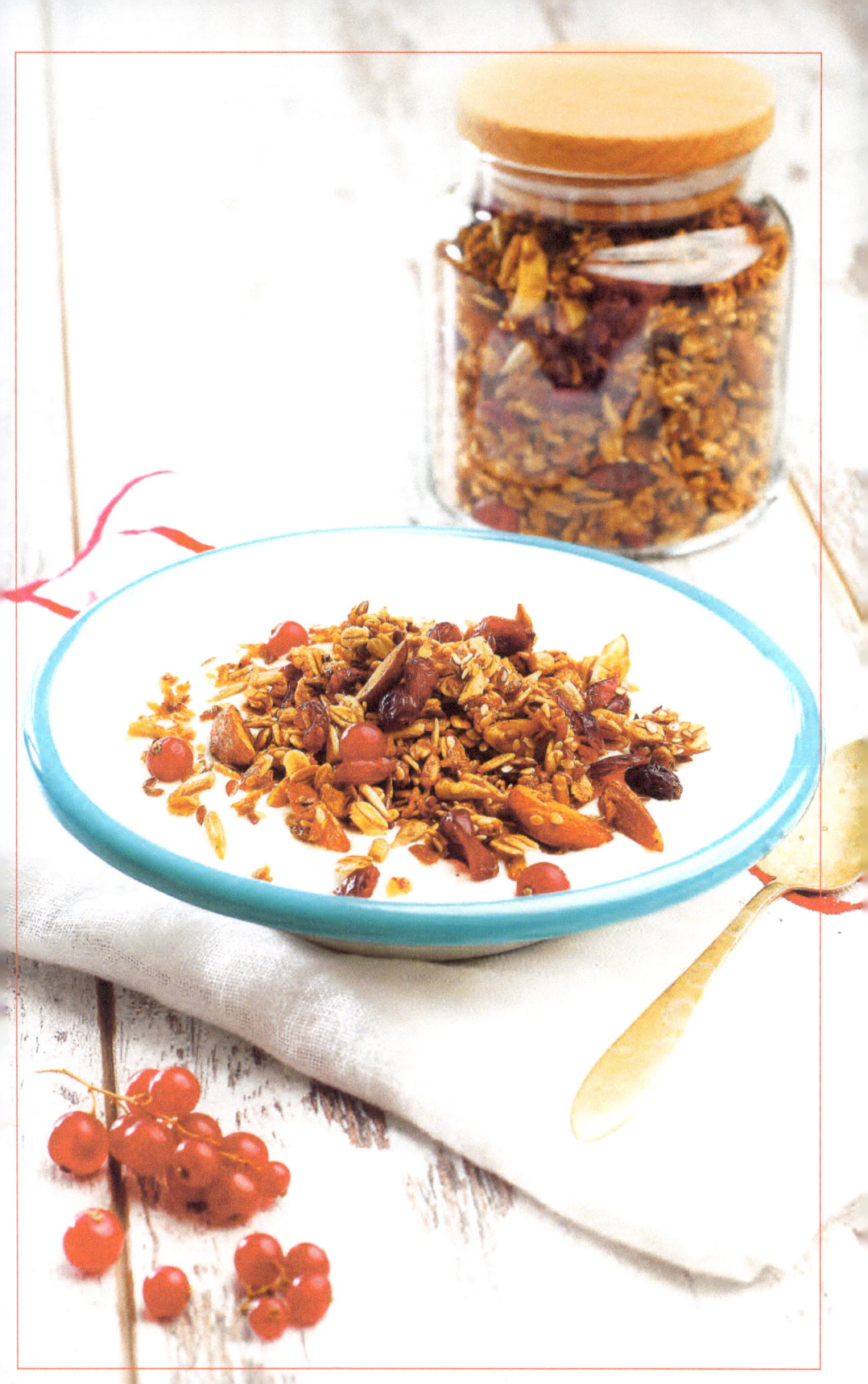

Pepper Shrimp

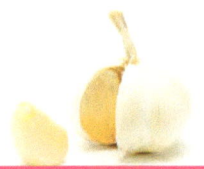

MAKES 3-4 SERVINGS

Ingredients

- 500g Shrimp, Peeled and Deveined
- Olive Oil
- 1 Sweet Red Pepper
- 3-4 Garlic Cloves
- Salt
- Crushed Red Pepper
- Water
- Fresh Ginger, Large Marble Size

Directions

1. Remove the seeds of the sweet red pepper and dice.
2. Grate the garlic.
3. Gently heat the olive oil in a skillet, add the garlic and slowly cook over medium heat.
4. Add the peeled and deveined shrimp, continuing to cook while stirring continuously.
5. Add 40ml of water, minced ginger, and sweet red pepper.
6. Season with salt and crushed red pepper to your taste; cook for 5 minutes, then serve.

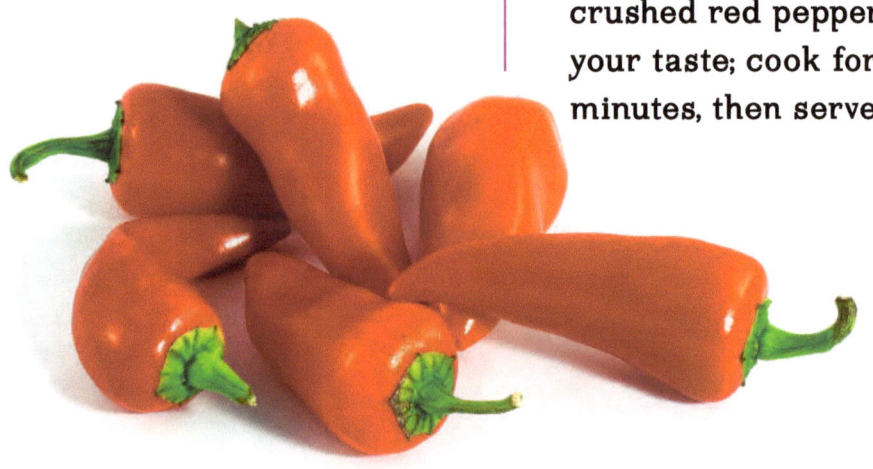

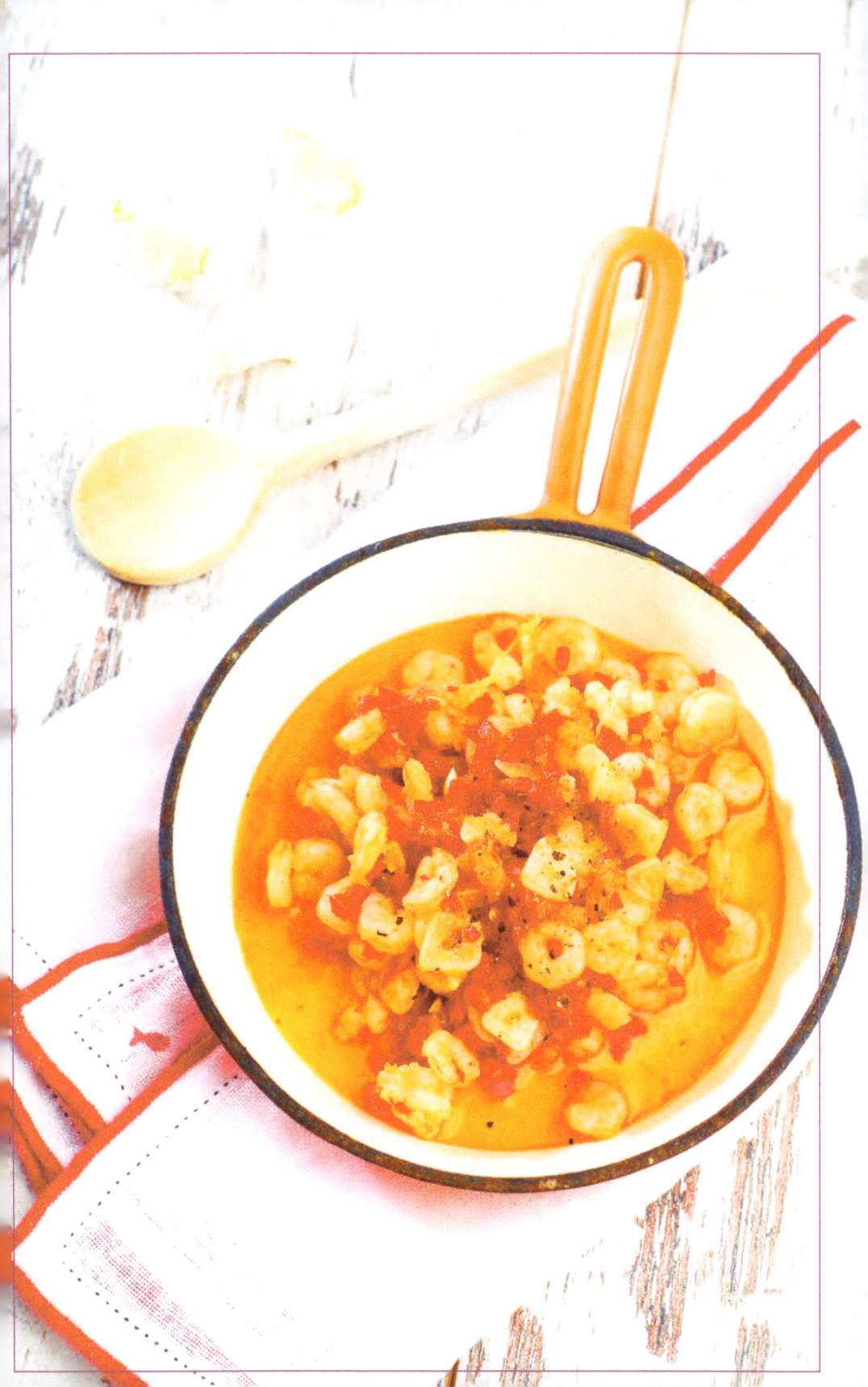

Spicy Lamb

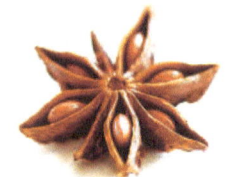

MAKES 2 SERVINGS

Ingredients

- 500g Leg of Lamb or Shank
- 1 Onion
- 1 Apple
- 1 Garlic Clove
- 1 Rosemary Sprig
- 3-4 Bay Leaves
- 8-10 Whole Black Peppercorns
- 3-4 Cardamom Pods
- 1 Whole Star Anise
- 2 Teaspoons Whole Coriander Seeds
- 1 Stick Cinnamon
- 5-6 Clove Pods
- 100ml Olive Oil
- 400ml Water

Directions

1. Peel the onion and cut into two halves.
2. Peel one clove of garlic and cut in half crosswise.
3. Add with all the other ingredients to a pressure cooker.
4. Cover and cook on high heat until it starts to whistle, then turn the heat to low and cook for 20 minutes.
5. If desired, serve with steamed vegetables on the side.

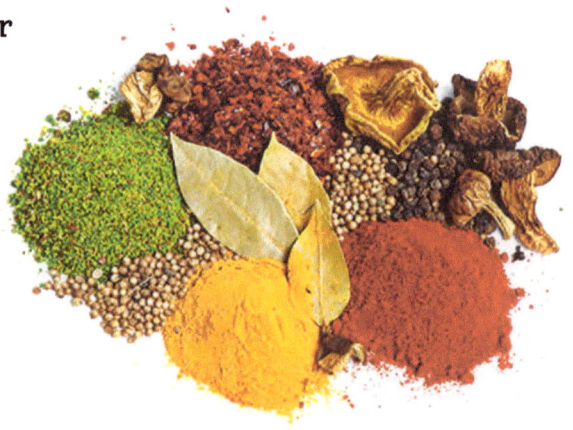

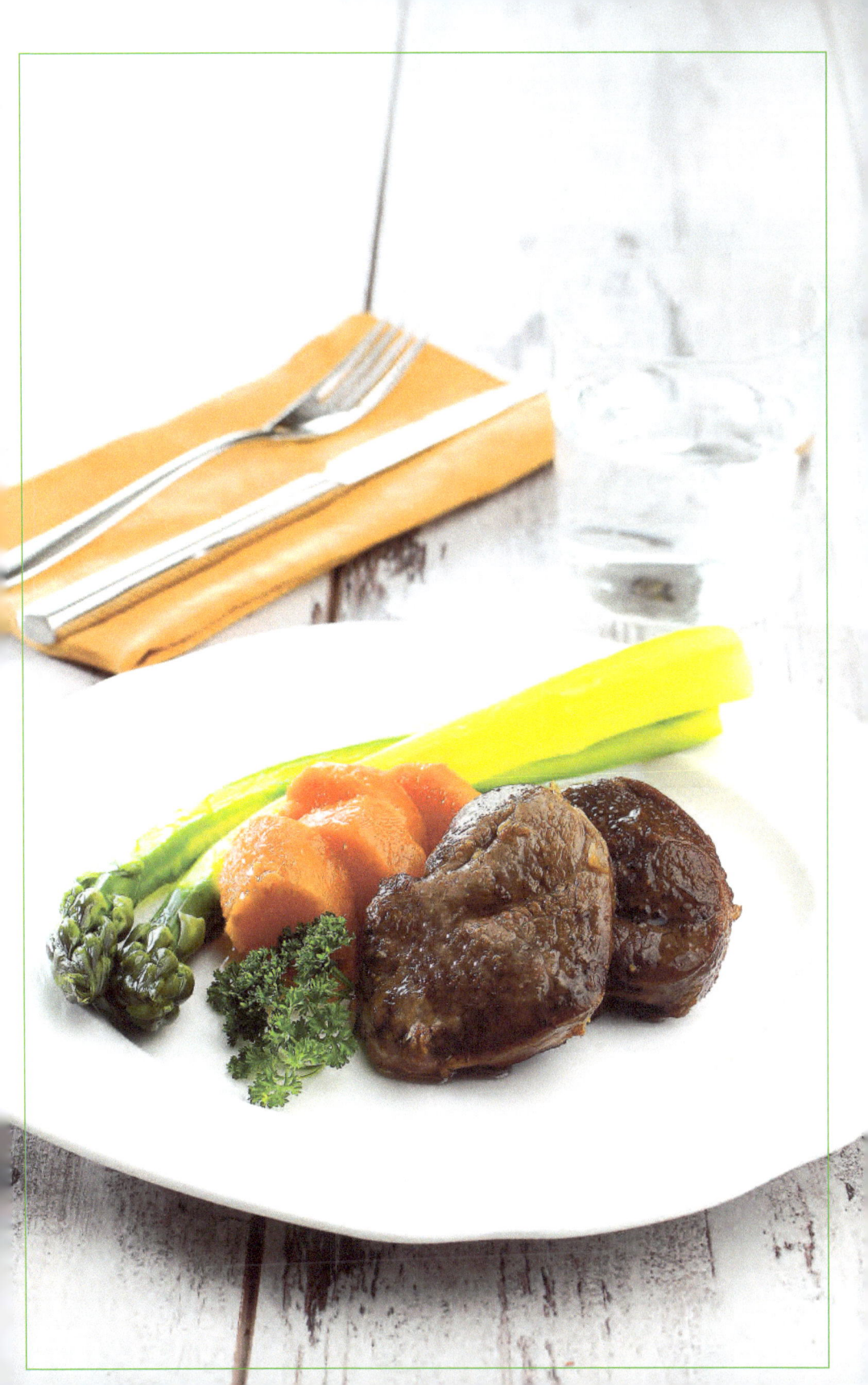

Sea Bass in Coconut Sauce

MAKES 2 SERVINGS

Ingredients

- 1 Sea Bass Fillet with Skin Removed
- 300ml Coconut Milk
- 1 Onion
- 3-4 Garlic Cloves
- Sea Salt
- Turmeric
- Cumin
- 1 Teaspoon Freshly Grated Ginger
- 10-15 Whole Black Peppercorns
- 2 Tablespoons Coconut Oil

Directions

1. Cut the onion into large chunks, add to the pan with peeled and sliced garlic and cook gently in a spoonful of coconut oil.
2. Add the coconut milk and spices. When it comes to a boil, turn off the heat.
3. Allow the sauce to cool for 10 minutes, then blend well in a blender.
4. Salt the fish and place it in a suitable baking pan with the remaining coconut oil.
5. Bake the fish at 200C for 10 minutes. If desired, you can boil two peeled and sliced potatoes for 10 minutes and add to the side of the fish before adding the sauce.
6. Pour the sauce over the fish and the potatoes, place the fish back in the oven, and cook for another 20-25 minutes.

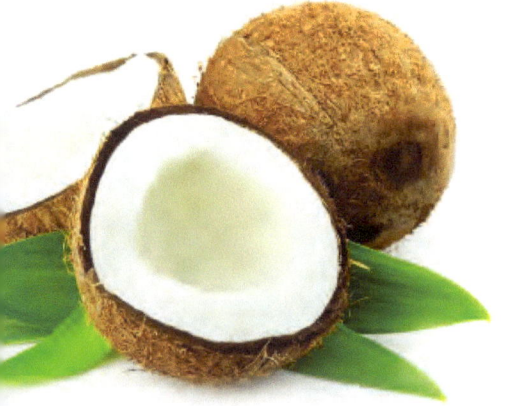

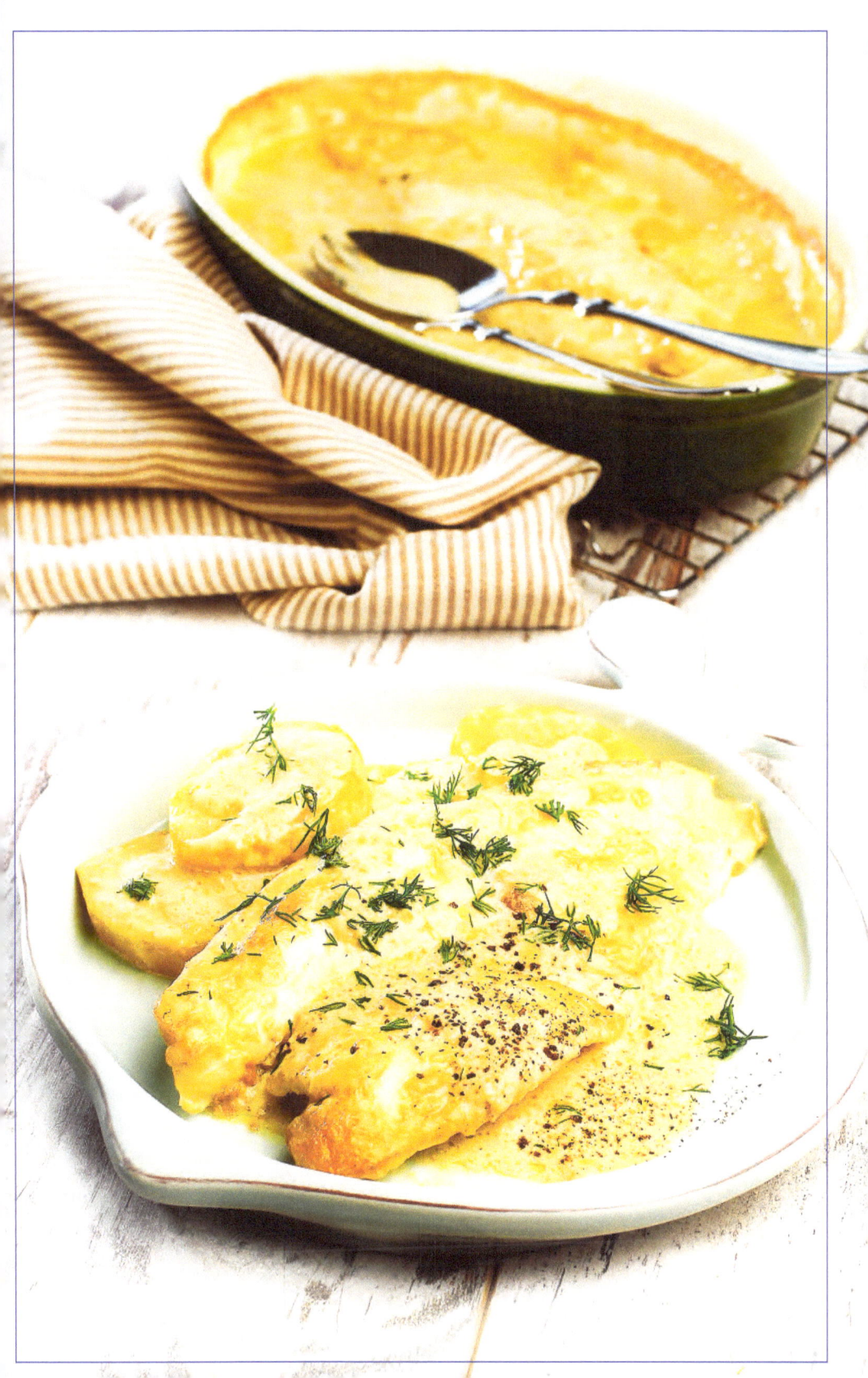

Pear Dessert

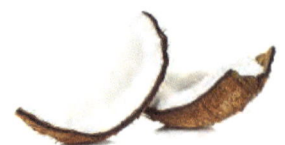

MAKES 2 SERVINGS

Ingredients

- 2 Pears
- 2 Tablespoons Grated Orange Zest
- 2 Dessertspoons Coconut Sugar
- 3-4 Cardamom Pods
- 1 Tablespoons Lemon Juice

Directions

1. Place the cardamom seeds in a mortar and crush them with a pestle.
2. Mix the cardamom, grated orange zest, coconut sugar and lemon juice in a bowl, adding an extra 1 or 2 spoons of water if needed.
3. Dip the peeled pears into the mixture and chill for half an hour.
4. Transfer the pears to a pot, add 200ml water, cook until pears become soft.
5. Serve with ice cream made of goat milk.
6. Note: If pears are sweet enough, you may not need to add sugar.

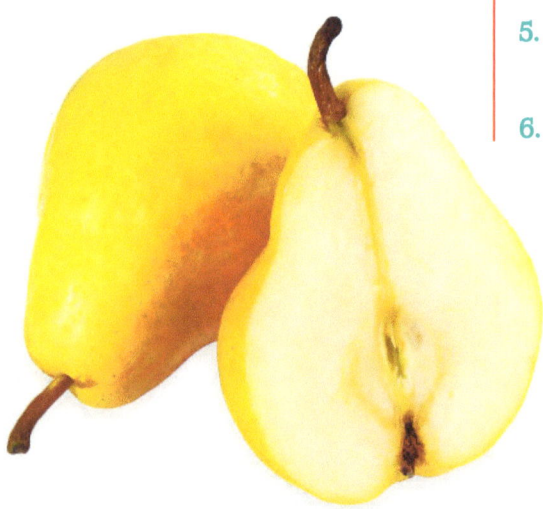

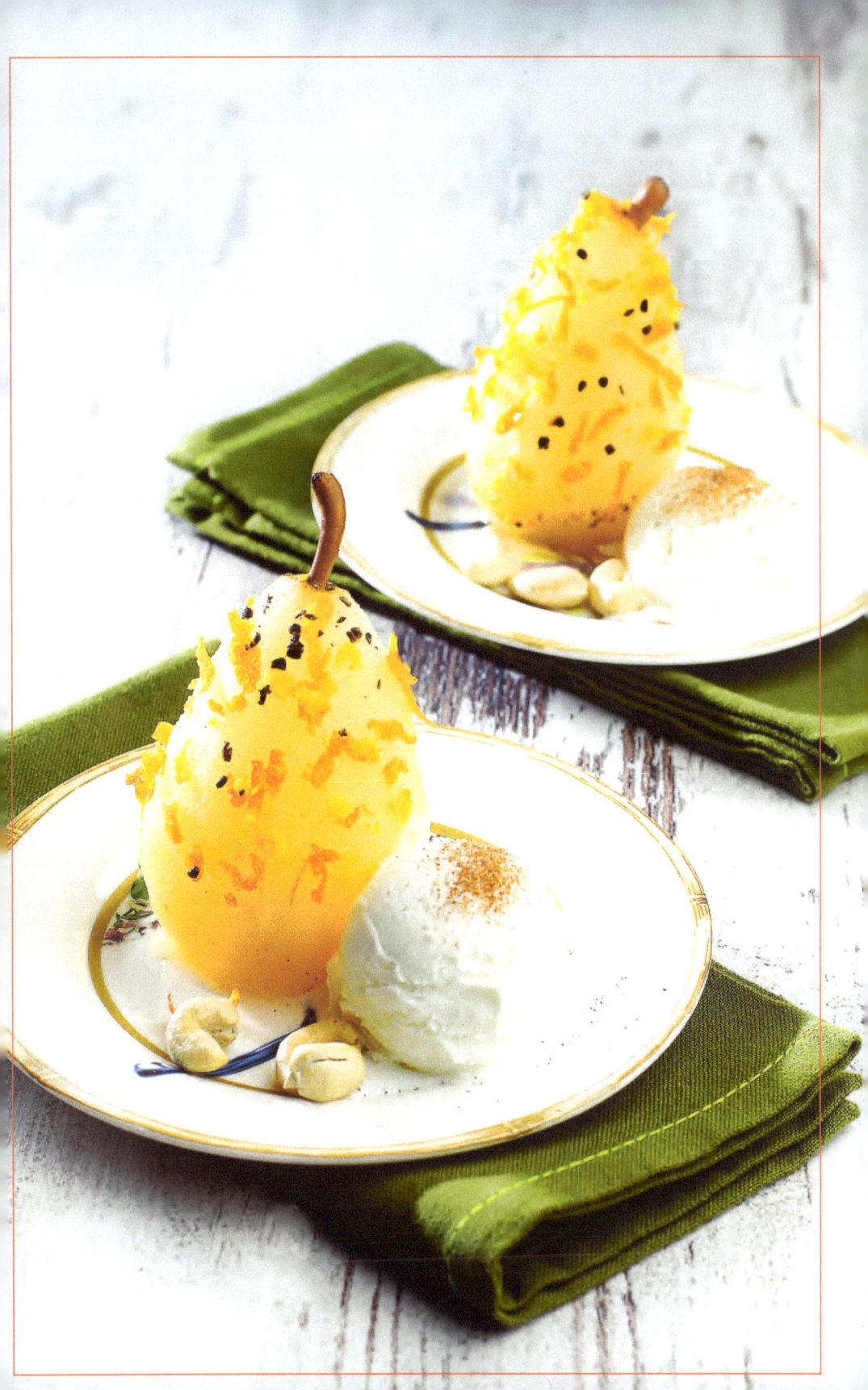

Strawberry Smoothie

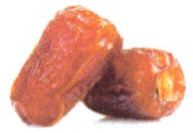

MAKES 2 SERVINGS

Ingredients

- 400ml Almond Milk
- 1 Bowl Strawberries
- 4-5 Dates
- 2 Teaspoon Maca Powder

Directions

1. Blend all ingredients in the blender until smooth, and then serve.

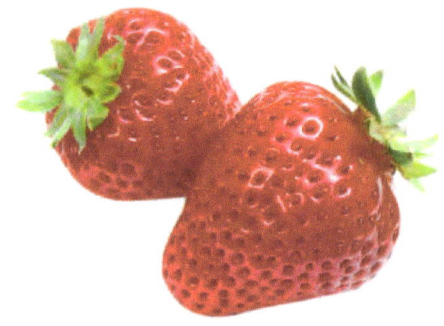

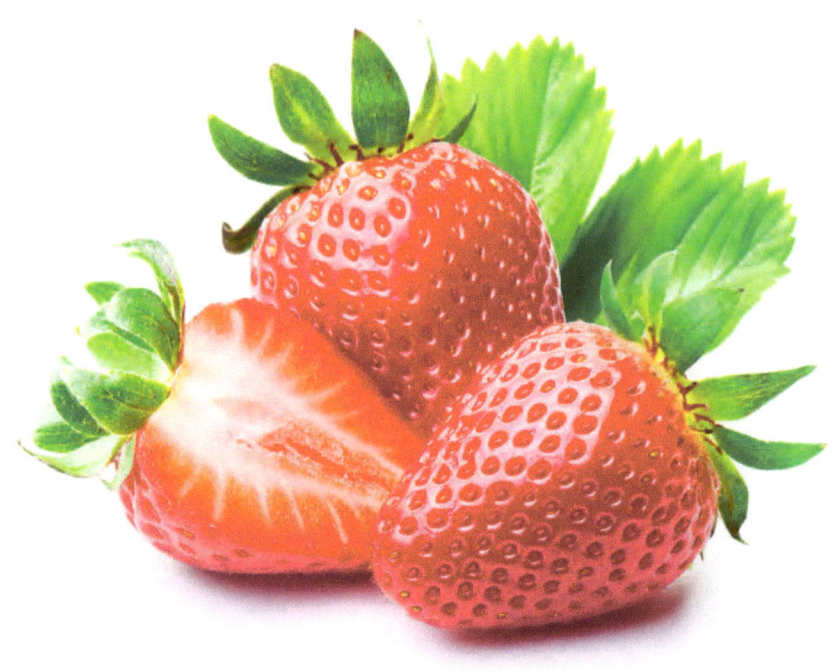

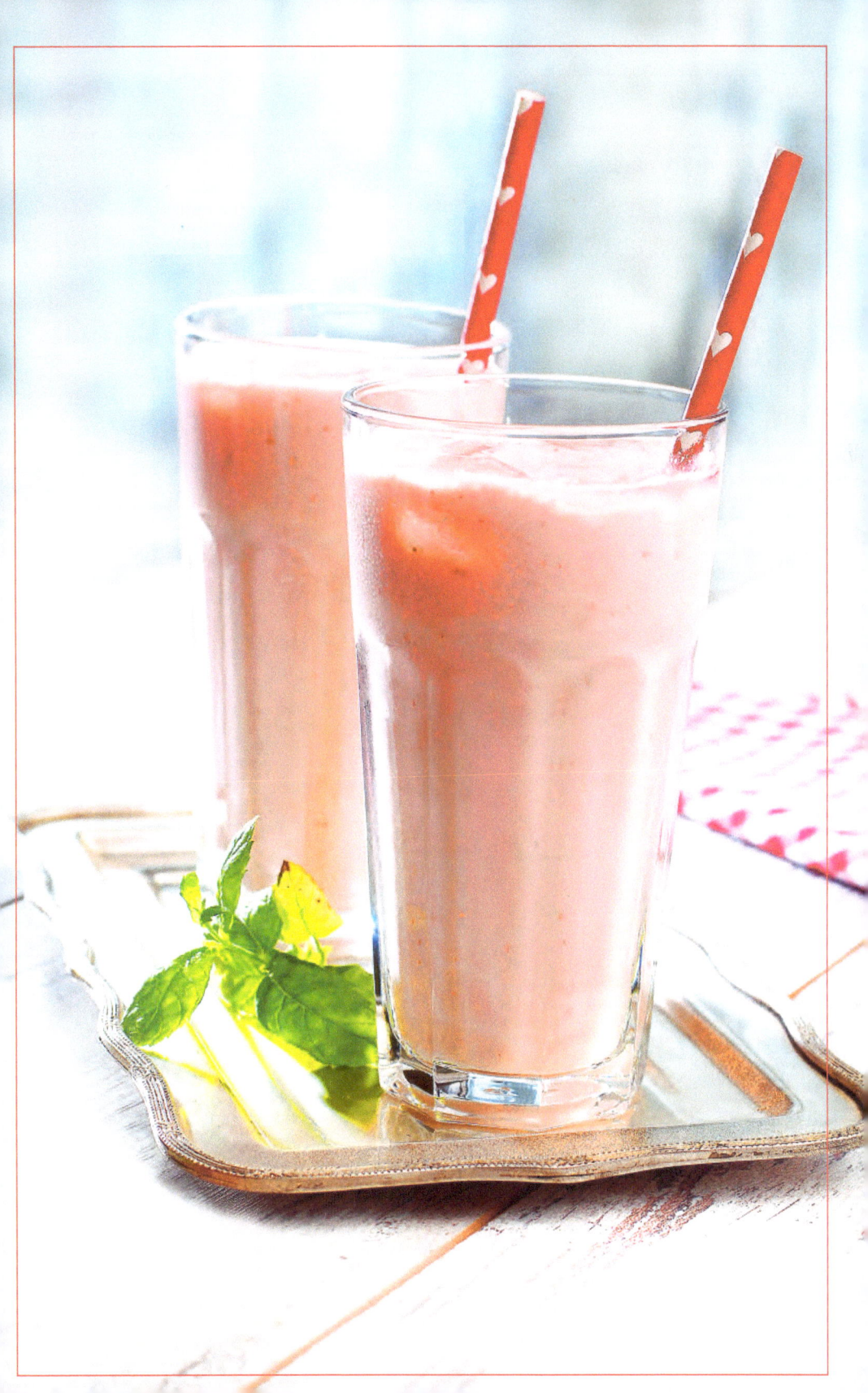

Coconut & Strawberry Coupe

MAKES 2 SERVINGS

Ingredients

- 1 Bowl Strawberries, Sliced and Whole
- 300ml Yogurt
- 3 Dessertspoons Freshly Grated Coconut
- 1 Teaspoon Maca Powder
- 2-3 Dessertspoons Coconut Sugar

Directions

1. Mix yogurt with coconut sugar, maca powder, and coconut thoroughly.
2. Divide half of the mixture between 2 serving cups.
3. Add the strawberries.
4. Pour the remaining mixture evenly over the strawberries.
5. Decorate with whole strawberries on top.
6. Serve cold.

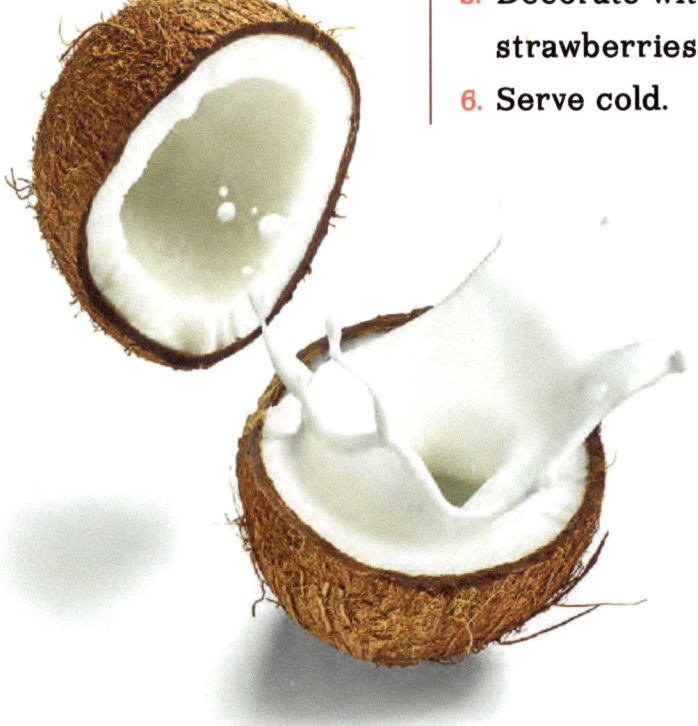

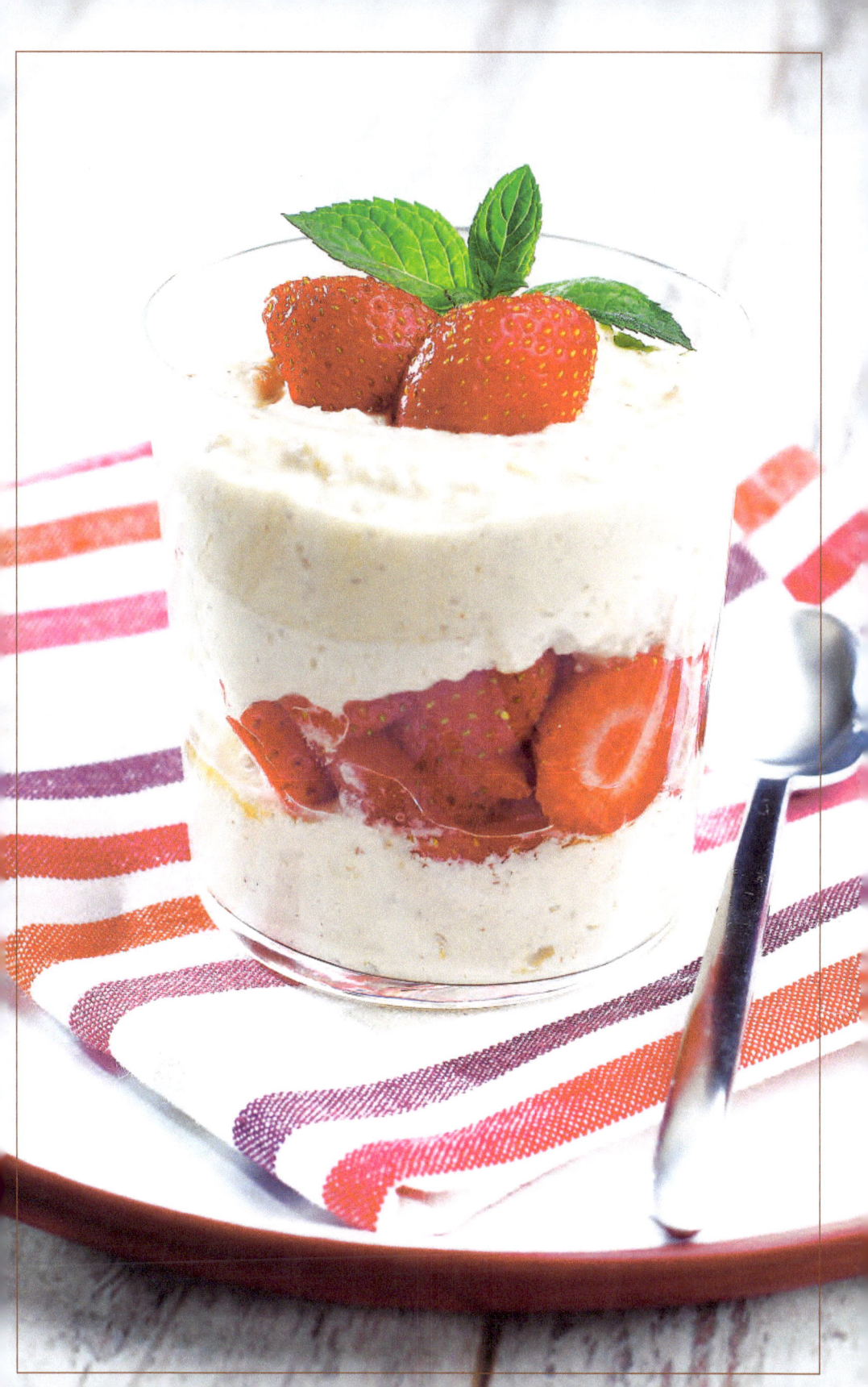

Root Vegetable Salad

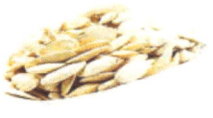

MAKES 5-6 SERVINGS

Ingredients

- 1 Red Beet
- 1 Carrot
- 1 Radish
- 1 Turnip Radish
- 1 Bowl Mediterranean Greens
- 1 Apple
- Pumpkin Seeds
- Salt
- 1 Dessertspoon Tahini
- Olive Oil
- Lemon

Directions

1. Wash the vegetables and grate them.
2. Wash the greens and slice the apples.
3. Combine all the ingredients in a salad bowl.
4. Thoroughly mix the olive oil, lemon juice, tahini and salt, then drizzle over the salad.
5. Toss to coat.
6. Toast pumpkin seeds and use as a garnish.

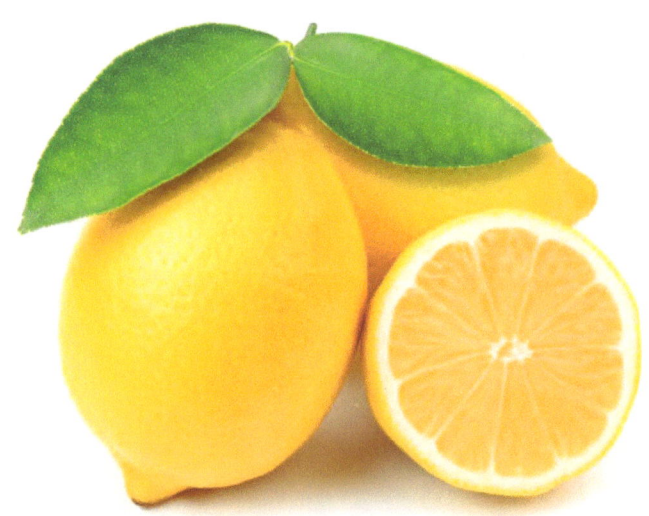

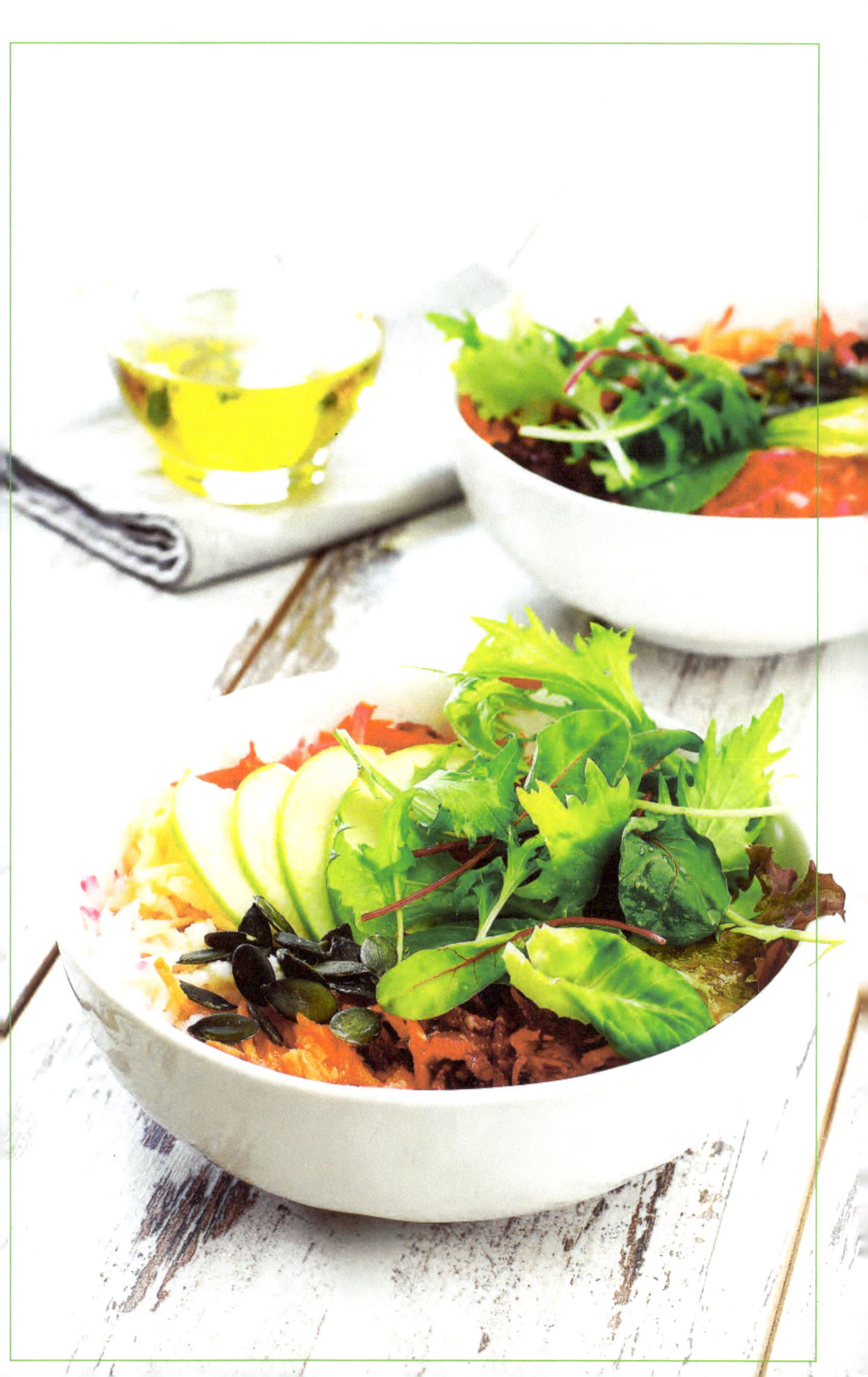

Nut Truffles

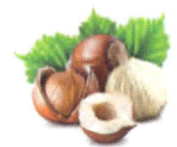

MAKES 7-8 SERVINGS

Ingredients

- 200ml Hazelnut-Walnut-Almond Mix
- 7-8 Cardamom Pods
- 100ml Raisins
- 10 Apricots
- 5 Dates
- 1 Tablespoon Cocoa

Topping

- 2-3 Tablespoons Shredded Coconut

Directions

1. Crush the cardamom in a mortar with a pestle.
2. Grind the hazelnut-walnut-almond mix, cardamom, raisins, apricots, dates, and cocoa together in a food processor.
3. Take small pieces of the mixture and roll them up into a ball shape.
4. Coat with shredded coconut and serve.

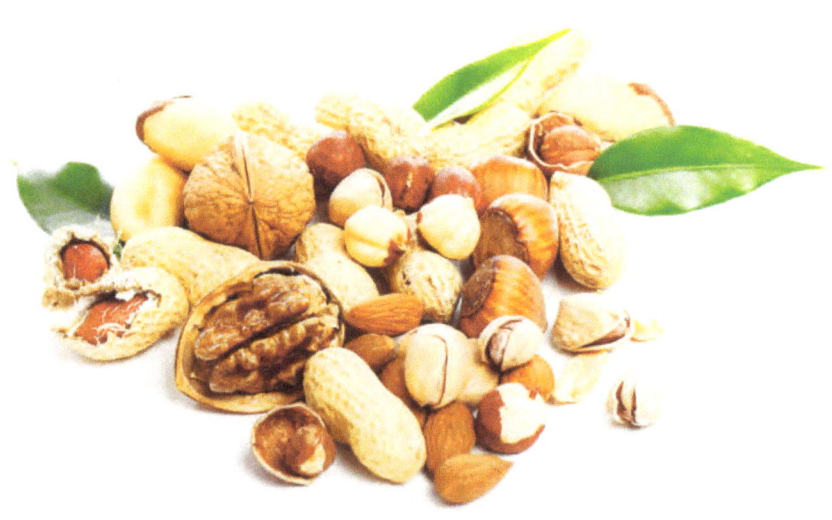

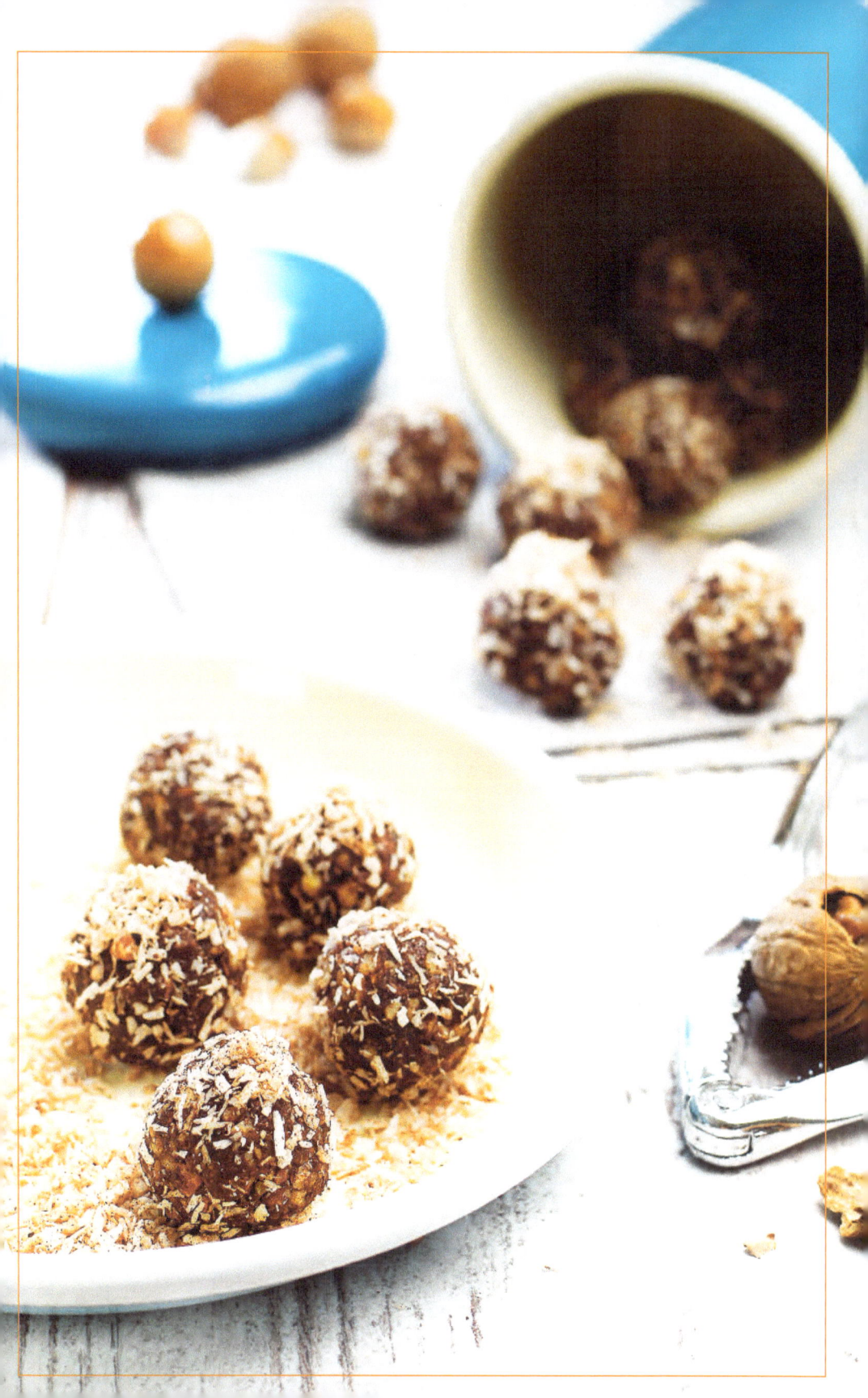

Fresh Fava Bean Puree

MAKES 4 SERVINGS

Ingredients

- 500g Fresh Fava Beans
- 1 Onion
- 3 Garlic Cloves
- Water
- 2-3 Tablespoons Olive Oil
- Salt
- Lemon
- Dill

Directions

1. Peel the outer skin off the fava beans. If beans are fresh you may skip the peeling process.
2. Remove the skin of the onion and cut into four pieces.
3. Peel the skin off the garlic.
4. Put the fresh fava beans, onion, and garlic cloves in a pot, and add water to cover.
5. Cook on high heat until the water comes to a boil, then turn the heat to low and cook until the fava beans are soft and tender.
6. Transfer the beans to a deep bowl after the water totally boils down and beans become mushy.
7. Season with olive oil, lemon juice and salt to taste, mash the beans to make a puree.
8. Decorate with dill and serve.

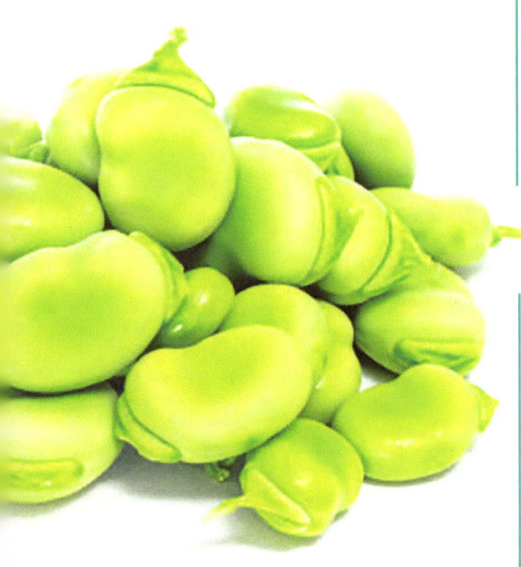

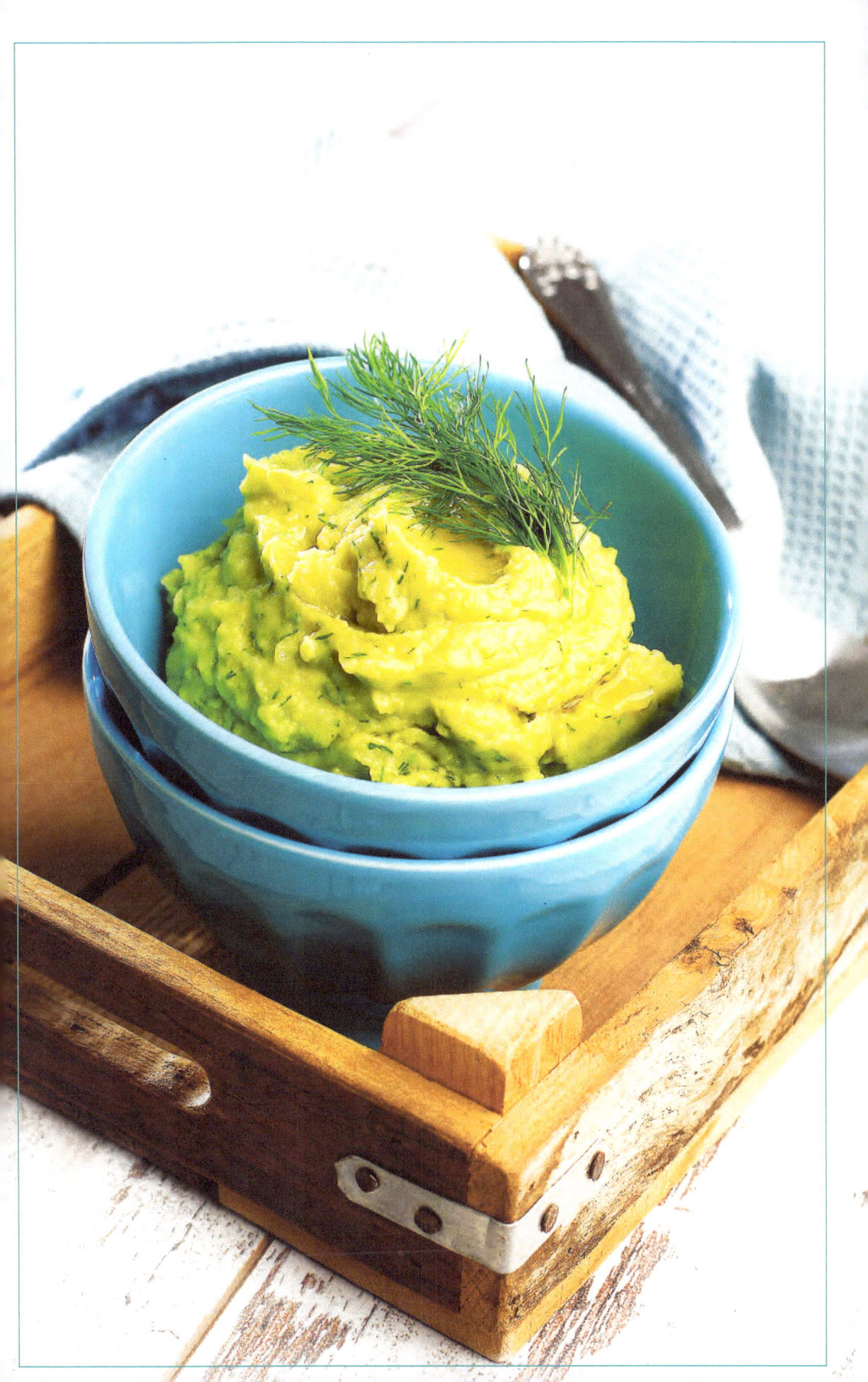

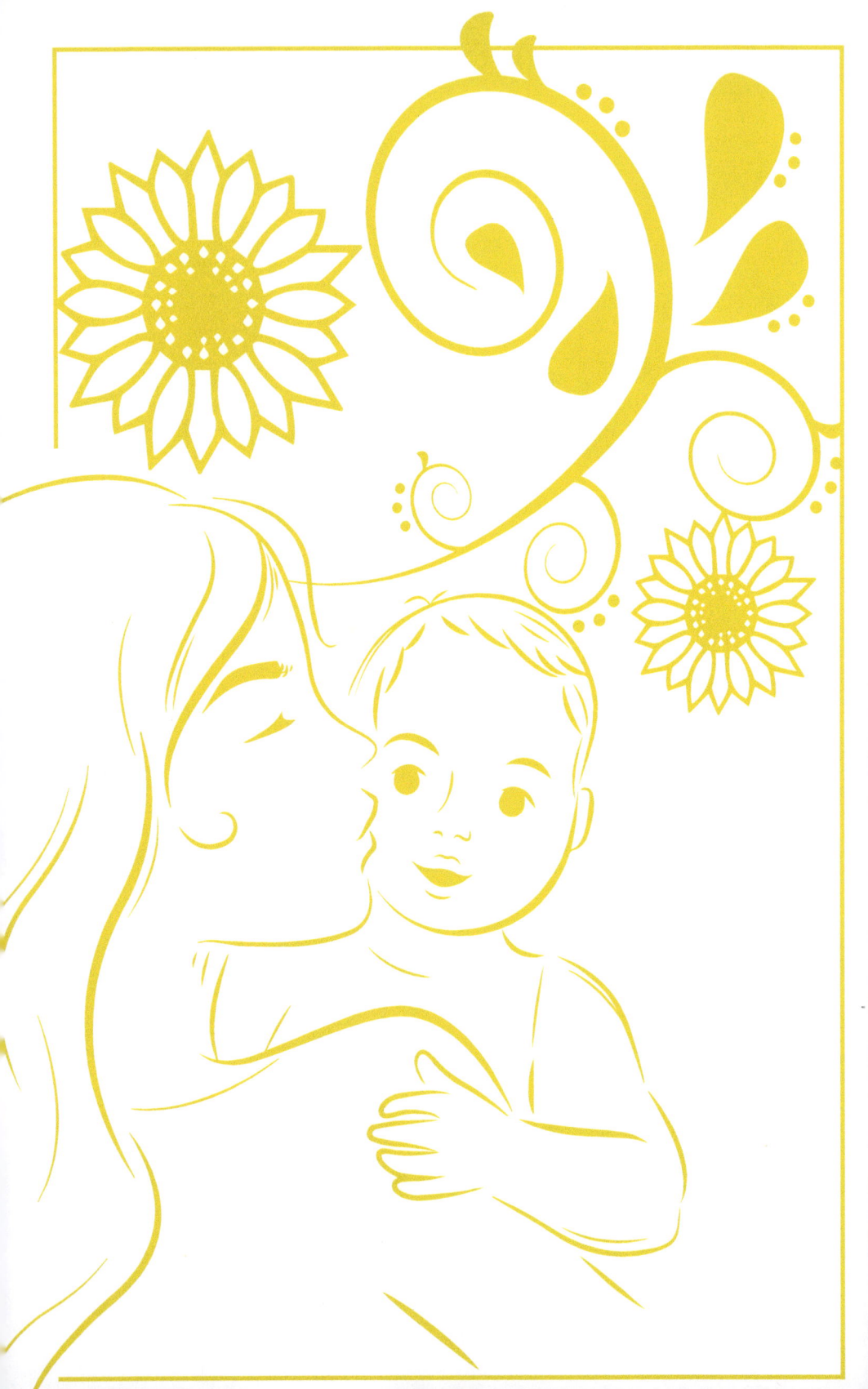

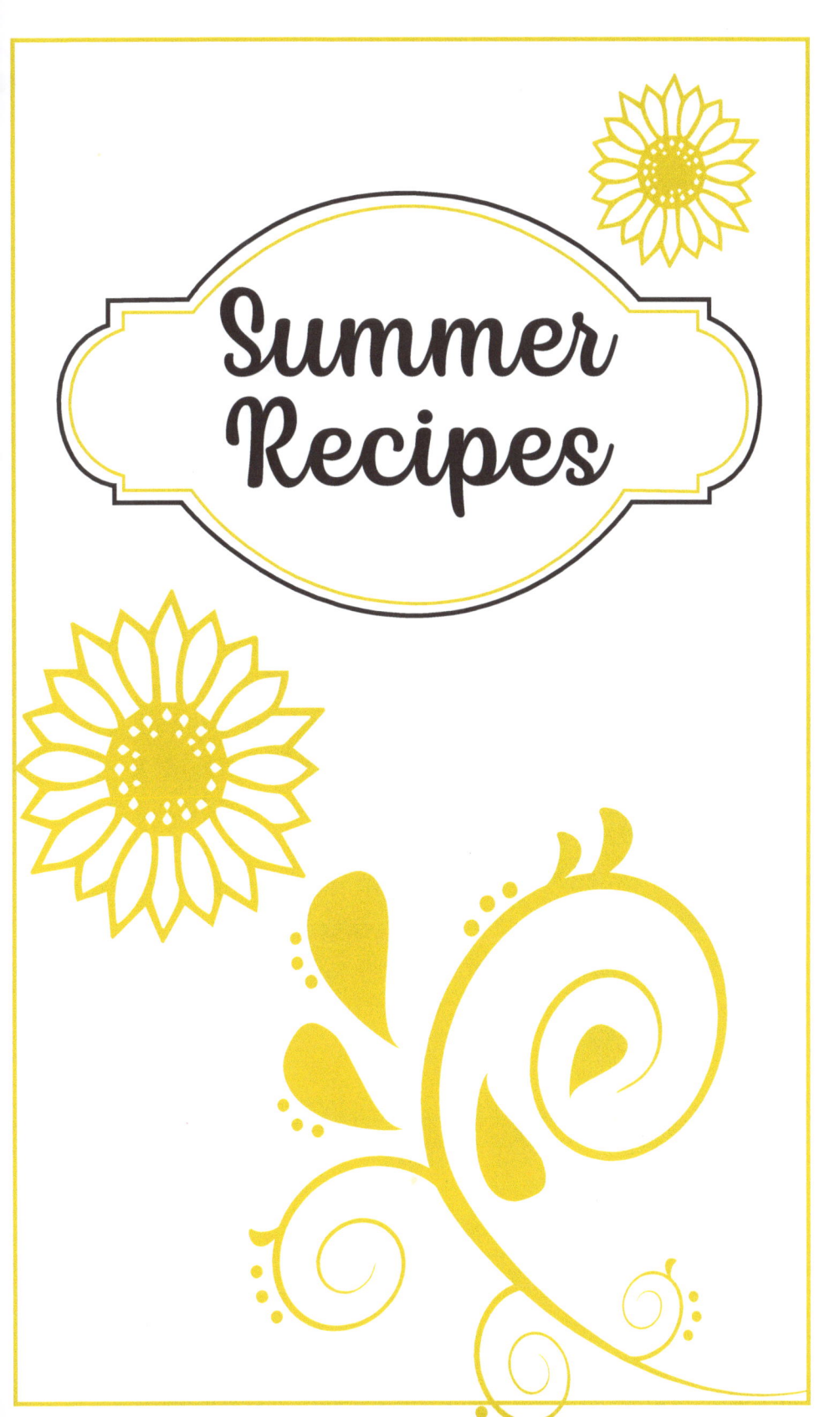

Avocado Salad

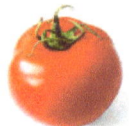

MAKES 3-4 SERVINGS

Ingredients

- 2 Avocados, Peeled and Pitted
- 1 Large Tomato
- 2 Cucumbers
- Parsley
- 3-4 Garlic Cloves
- Lemon
- Olive Oil

Directions

1. Set a quarter of an avocado aside. Dice the remaining avocados, tomato, and cucumbers.
2. Mince the parsley.
3. Combine all the ingredients in a bowl.
4. Grate the garlic, and mix with olive oil and lemon juice; add the quarter piece of avocado and blend into the sauce by mashing with a fork. Add salt to taste. Pour over the salad.
5. Chill for 30 minutes before serving.

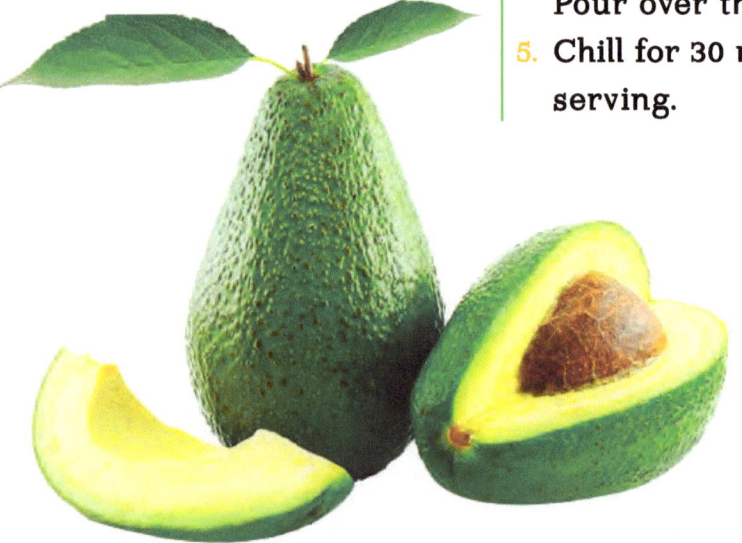

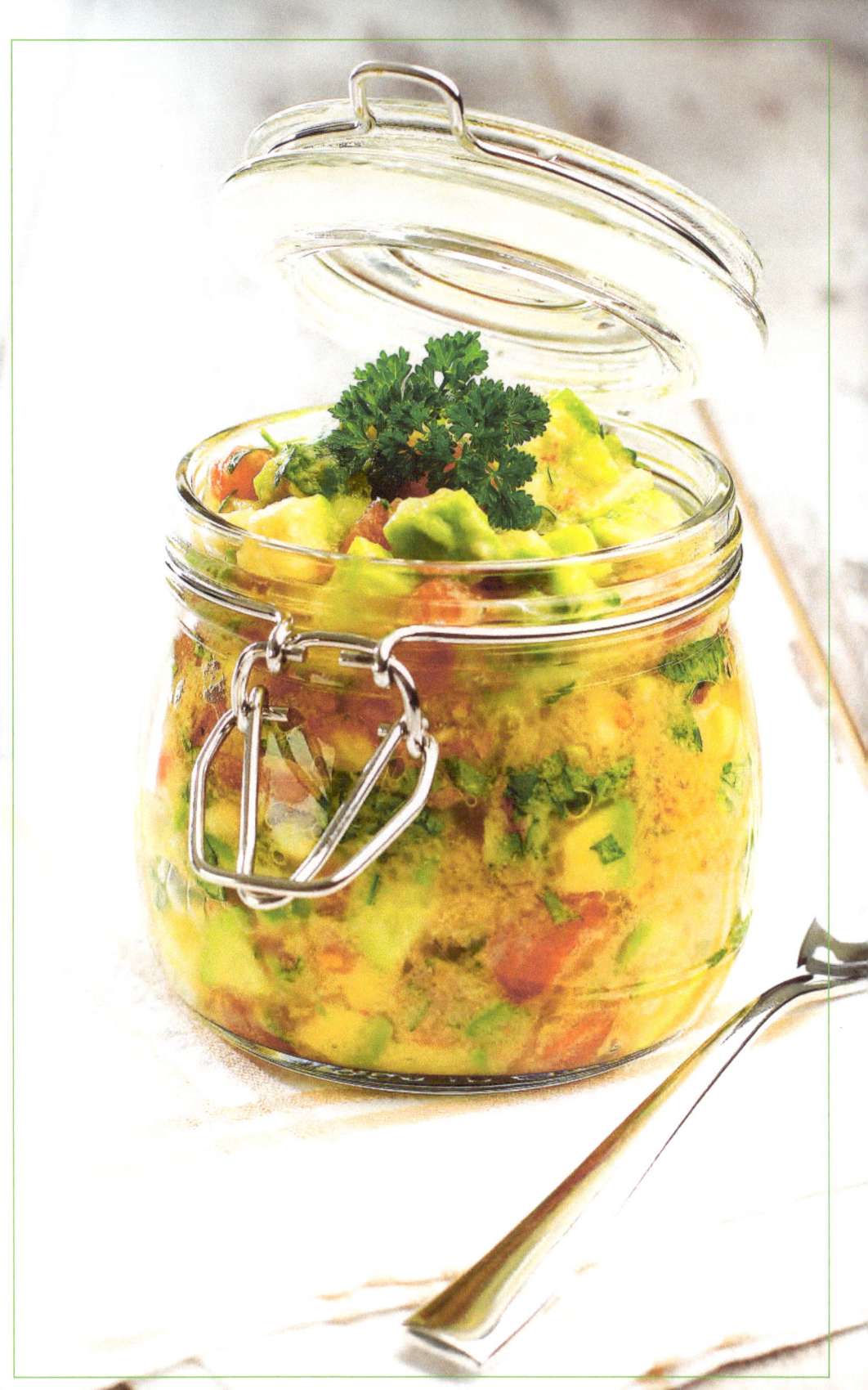

Chia, Raspberry & Kefir Smoothie

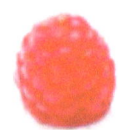

MAKES 2 SERVINGS

Ingredients

- 300ml Kefir
- 1 Banana (preferably from Anamur)
- 100ml Raspberries
- 1 Tablespoon Chia Seeds

Directions

1. Peel the banana and put in a blender.
2. Add kefir, raspberries, and chia seeds and blend until smooth.
3. Pour into glasses and serve immediately.

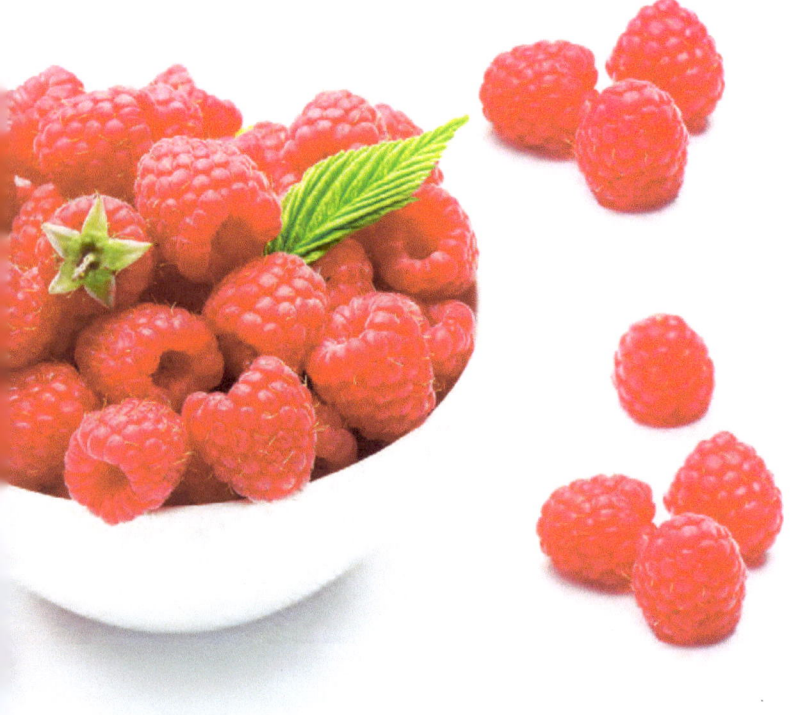

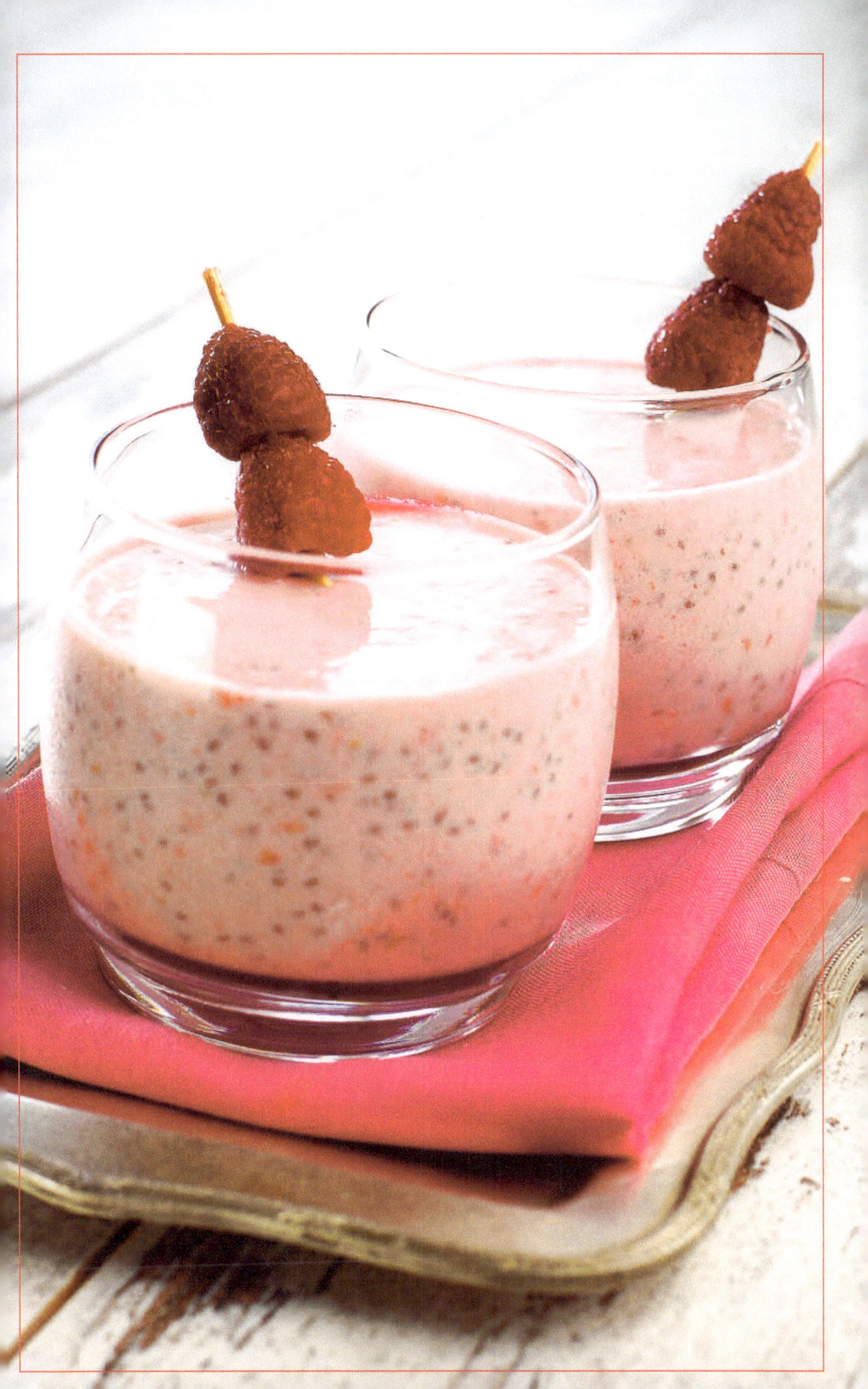

Chia Pudding

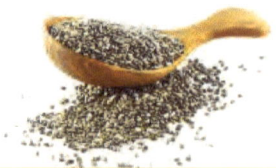

MAKES 4-5 SERVINGS

Ingredients

- 400ml Coconut Milk
- 400ml Water
- 5 Sticks Cinnamon
- 4-5 Clove Pods
- 2 Tablespoons Coconut Sugar
- 130ml Chia Seeds
- 2-3 Tablespoons Cranberries
- Mixed Fruits for Garnishing

Directions

1. Place milk, water, cinnamon sticks, and clove pods in a medium-size saucepan and heat over medium heat just until mixture comes to a boil.
2. Then turn the heat to low and let simmer for 15 minutes.
3. Turn the heat off and allow to cool for 10 minutes.
4. Strain through a sieve.
5. Add coconut sugar, cranberries, and chia seeds to the liquid and stir gently, making sure there are no lumps.
6. Pour the pudding into serving cups.
7. Chill 3 or 4 hours.
8. Decorate with mixed seasonal fruits and serve.

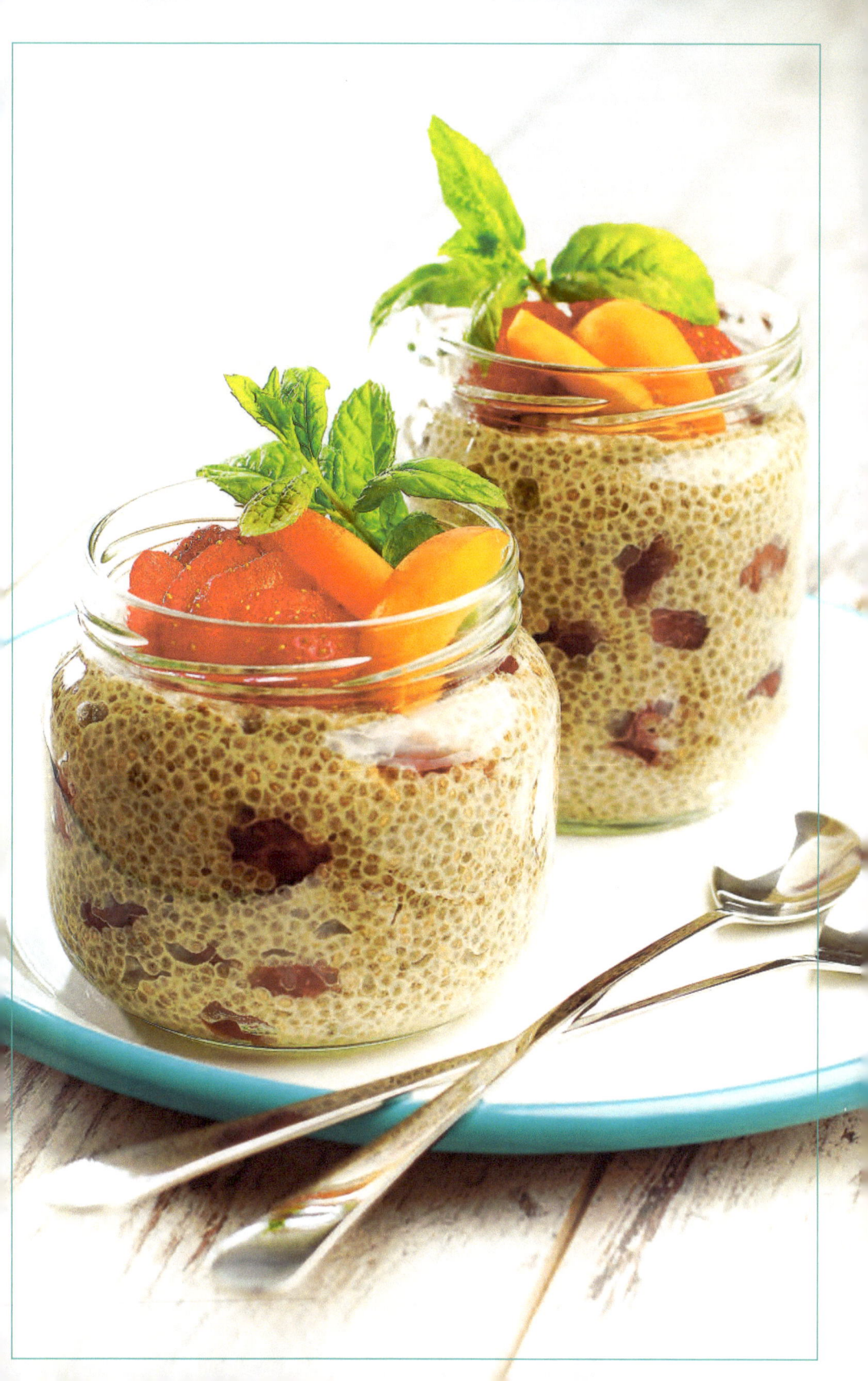

Strawberry Ice Cream

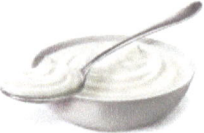

MAKES 3-4 SERVINGS

Ingredients

- ½ kg Strawberries
- 2 Tablespoons Coconut Sugar
- ½ Tablespoons Lemon Juice
- 400ml Condensed Yogurt

Directions

1. Wash and clean strawberries. Mix with coconut sugar and lemon juice, and chill in the refrigerator for 1 or 2 hours.
2. Blend the strawberries with the condensed yogurt in a blender.
3. Place the mixture in a freezer.
4. After 40 minutes, remove from the freezer and blend it again. Repeat this process 4 or 5 times.
5. Finally, pour into a suitable container and let it freeze.
6. Use a scoop to make ice cream balls. The ice cream can be served with other fruits if desired.

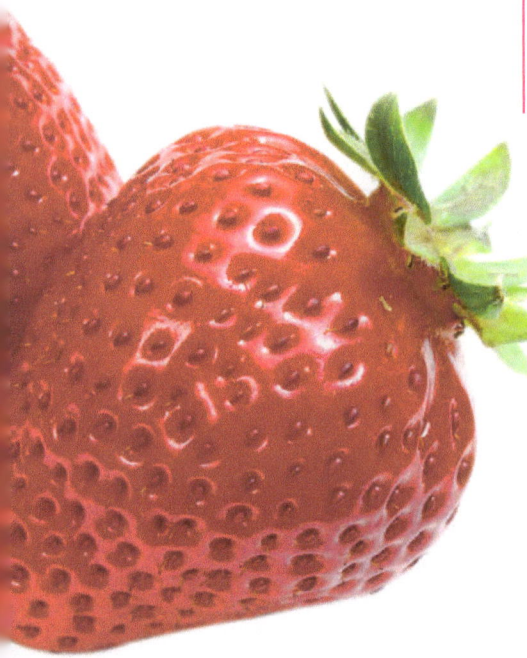

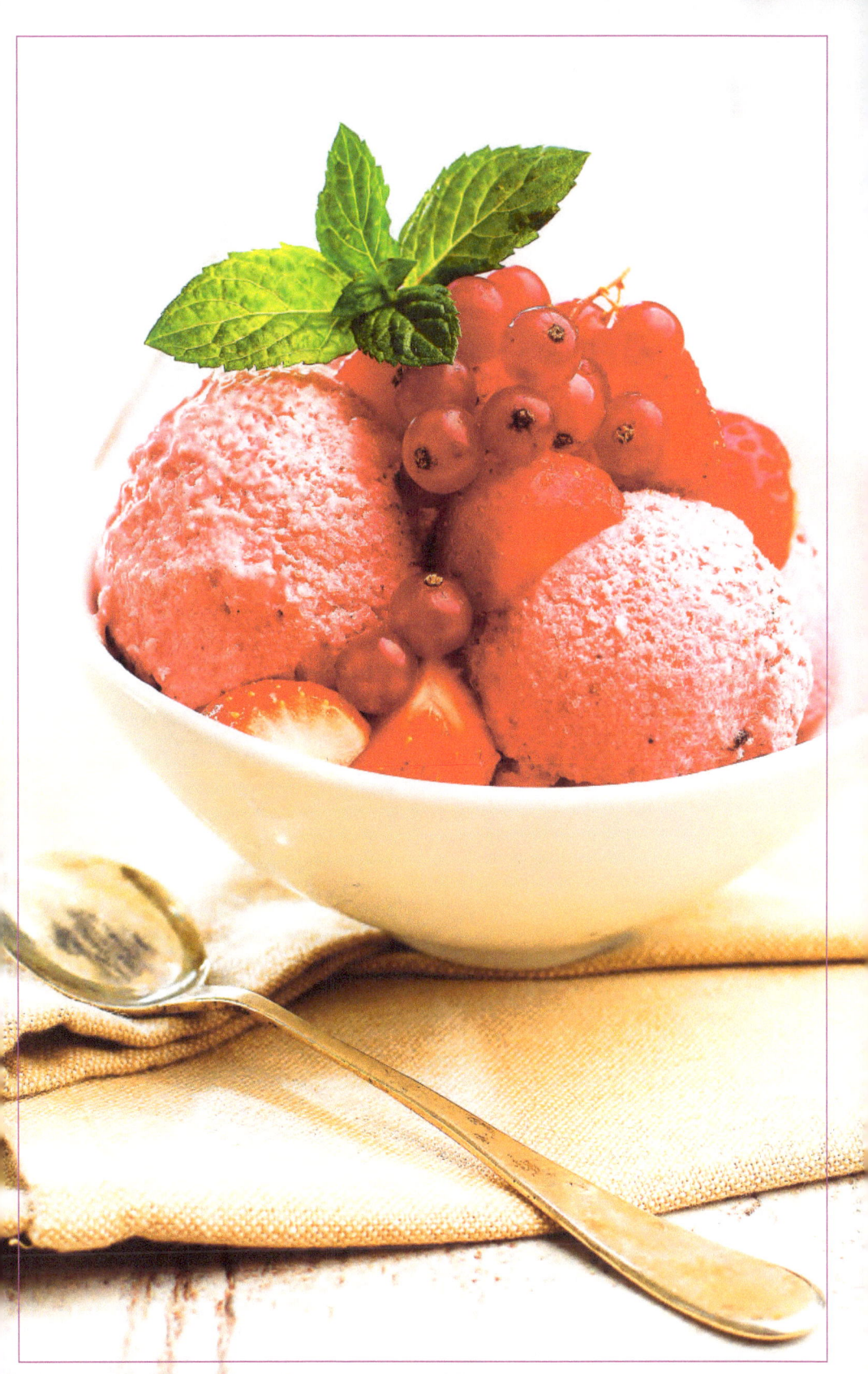

Sea Asparagus (Samfir) with Garlic

MAKES 6-8 SERVINGS

Ingredients

- 2 Bunches of Sea Asparagus
- 1 Lemon
- 100ml Olive Oil
- 4 Garlic Cloves
- Chopped Walnuts

Directions

1. Soak the sea asparagus in a pot of water for an hour.
2. Drain the sea asparagus spears, and wash them one by one.
3. Bring a large pot of water to boil. Add the sea asparagus and cook for 15 minutes.
4. Prepare a large bowl of ice water. With a spatula, transfer the asparagus to the ice water.
5. Grab the asparagus at the root with one hand and slide the green part off the stem with your other hand.
6. Blend garlic, olive oil and lemon juice in a blender to create a simple sauce.
7. Drizzle over the sea asparagus and toss to coat.
8. Serve with crumbled walnuts over top.

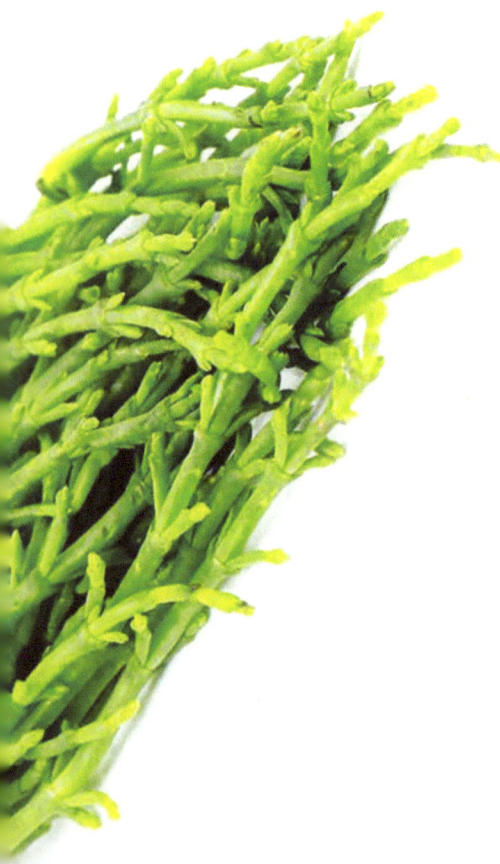

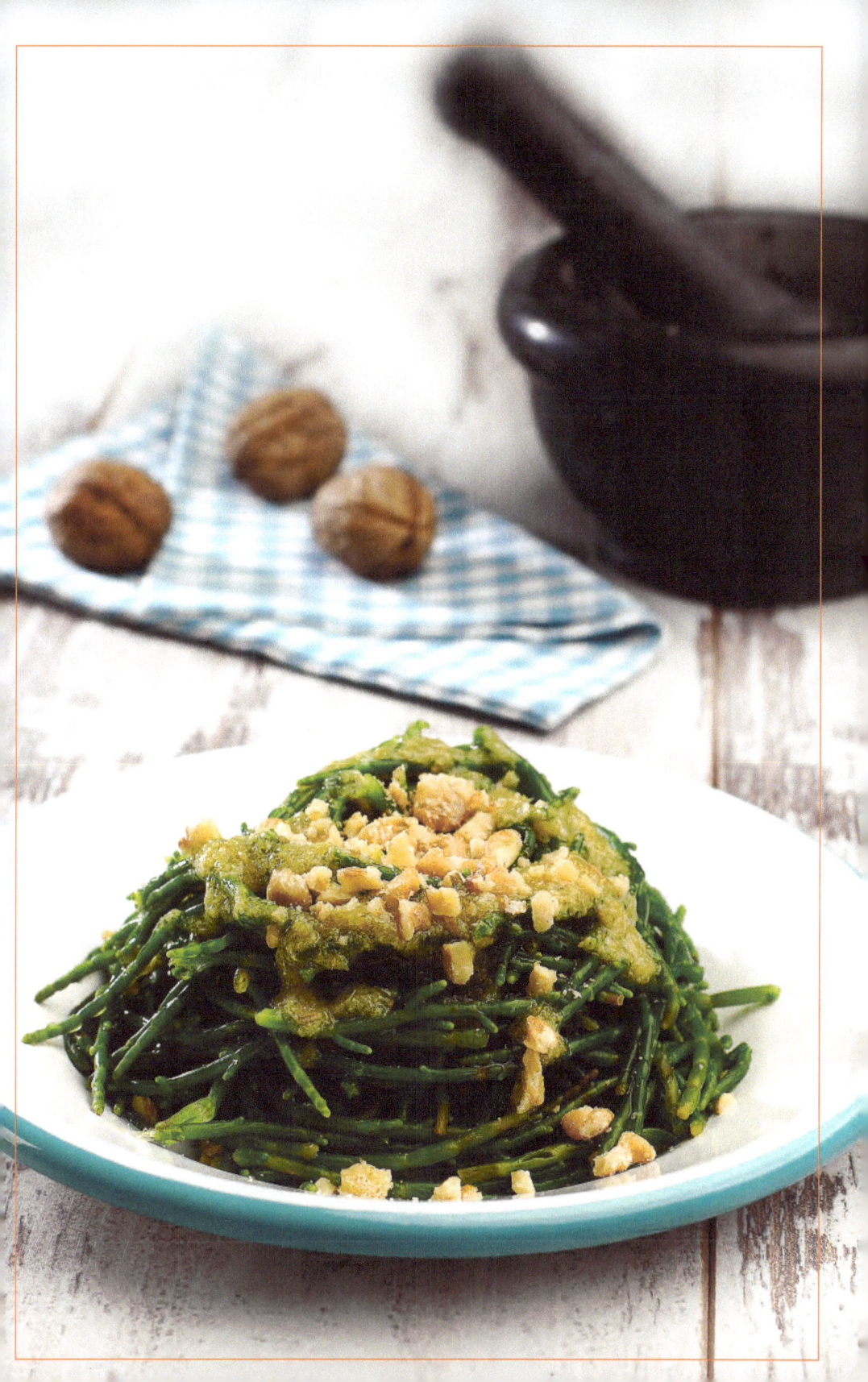

Stuffed Peppers with Ground Beef

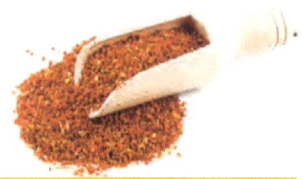

MAKES 6-8 SERVINGS

Ingredients

- 10-15 Bell Peppers
- 250g Ground Beef
- 200ml Siyez (Einkorn) Bulgur
- 2 Onions
- 2 Tomatoes, Finely Chopped
- 1 Tablespoons Tomato Paste
- Parsley
- Salt
- Black Pepper
- Crushed Red Pepper
- Olive Oil
- 1 Tomato to Cap the Bell Peppers

Sauce

- 1 Tablespoon Tomato Paste

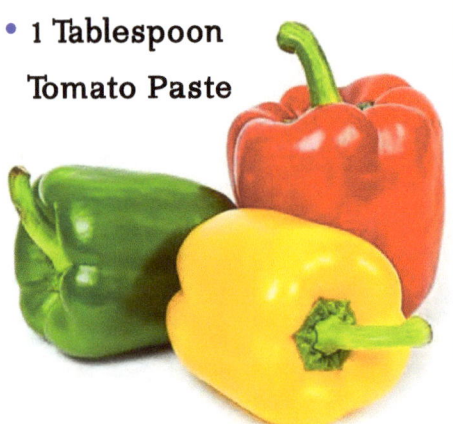

Directions

1. Wash, core, and seed the bell peppers. Let them drain in a colander.
2. Cook the diced onions in olive oil over medium heat.
3. Add the ground beef, stirring continuously, and cook until it gives out its juice and absorbs it back.
4. Add the tomatoes, tomato paste, salt, black pepper and red pepper.
6. Add the washed and drained Siyez bulgur and minced parsley last. Turn off heat and allow it to cool.
7. Pack the peppers with the filling, and use tomato pieces to cap the peppers.
8. Mix the tomato paste with a little hot water to prepare a sauce, and pour over the stuffed peppers. Add water to the pot to cover half of the peppers.
9. Cook on medium heat until it comes to a boil, then turn the heat to low. Cook until the peppers and the bulgur are soft.

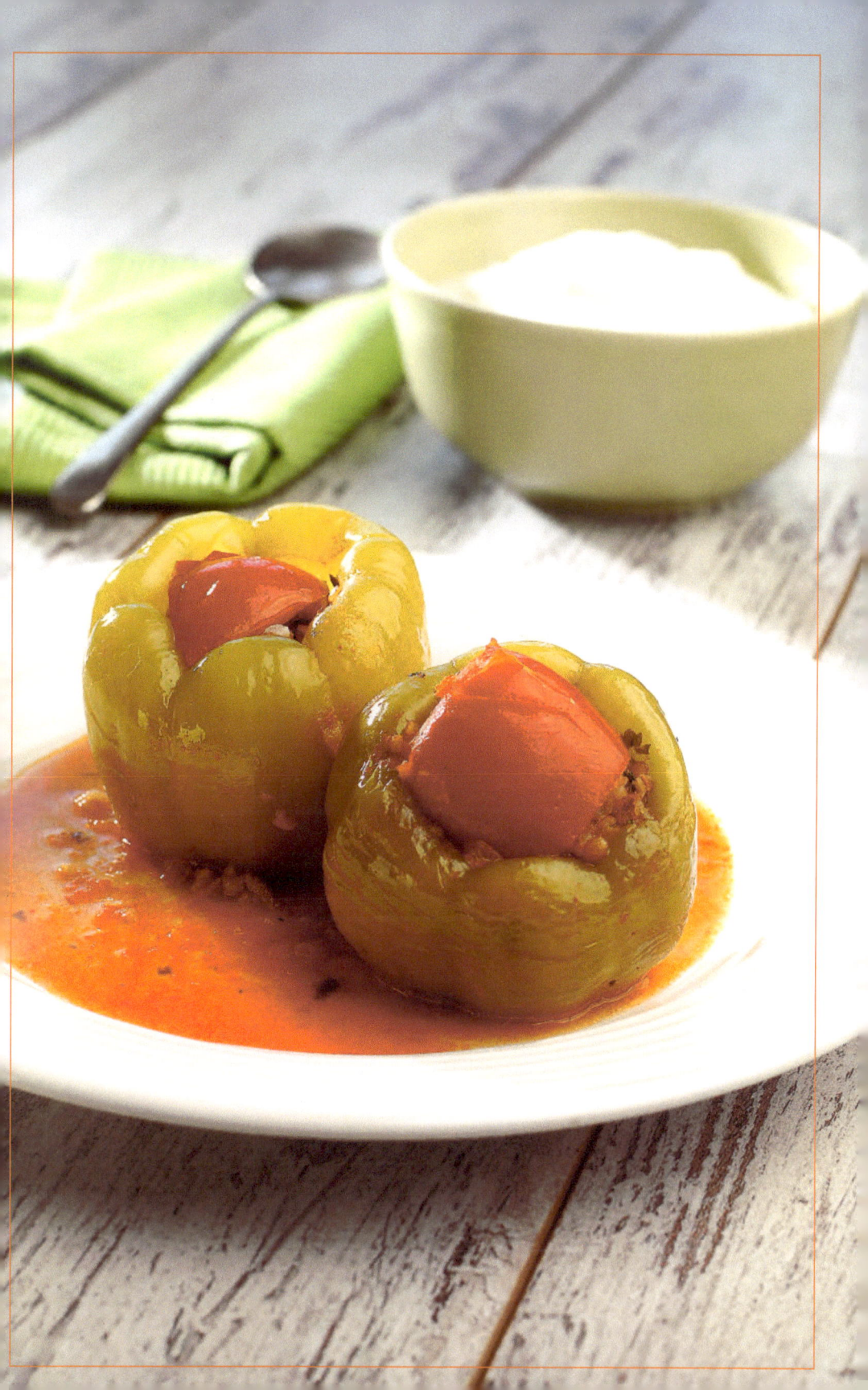

Hazelnut or Almond Butter

MAKES 7-8 SERVINGS

Ingredients

- ½ Kilogram Raw Hazelnuts or Almonds
- ½ Vanilla Pod (scrape out seeds)
- 6-7 Cardamom Pods

Directions

1. Combine raw hazelnuts or almonds with scraped vanilla seeds and cardamom in a food processor and chop at high speed.
2. Since hazelnuts are oily, they will reach a creamy texture faster than almonds.
3. Stop your food processor from time to time to scrape the mass that forms on the sides with a knife.
4. For better consistency with almonds, you can add a tablespoon of coconut oil to the mixture.
5. Stored in a clean mason jar in the refrigerator, butter will stay fresh for a long time.

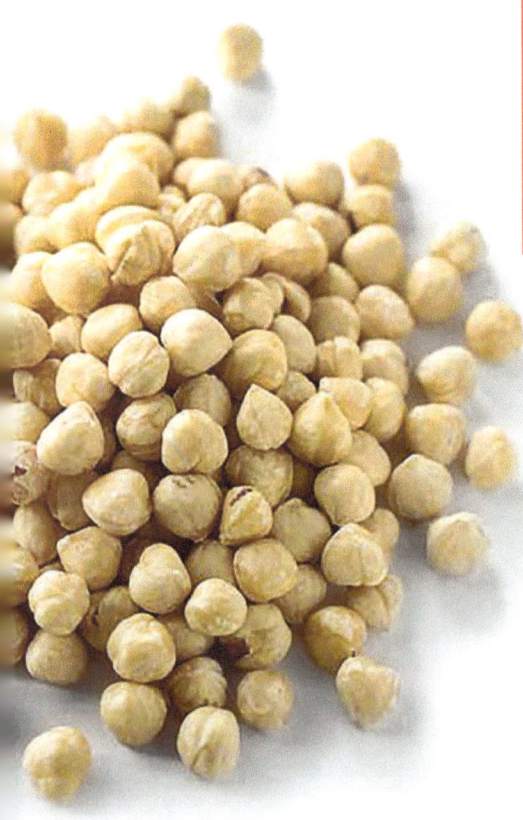

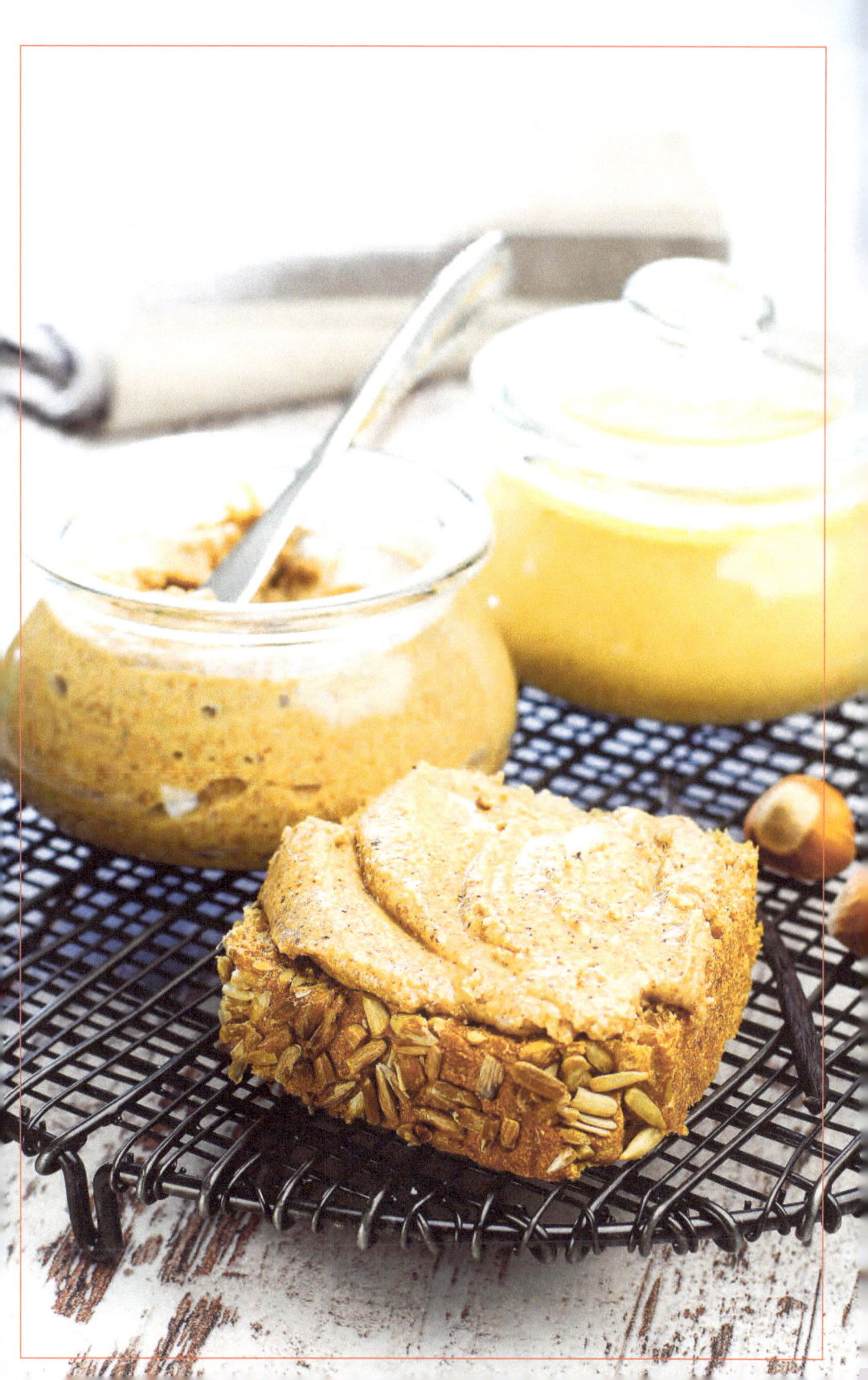

Oven Roasted Vegetables

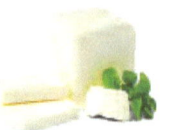

MAKES 4 SERVINGS

Ingredients

- 2 Zucchini
- 2 Carrots
- 2 Sweet Red Peppers
- 1 Onion
- 2-3 Fresh Garlic Cloves
- Fresh Mint, Rosemary, Thyme
- Sea Salt
- Extra Virgin Olive Oil
- 1 Small Piece Fresh Ginger
- Goat Cheese

Directions

1. Wash and slice the vegetables.
2. Clean and mince the herbs.
3. Chop the garlic and ginger.
4. Mix all the ingredients and spread evenly in a roasting pan.
5. Preheat the oven to 200C.
6. Roast until all vegetables are tender. Serve warm.

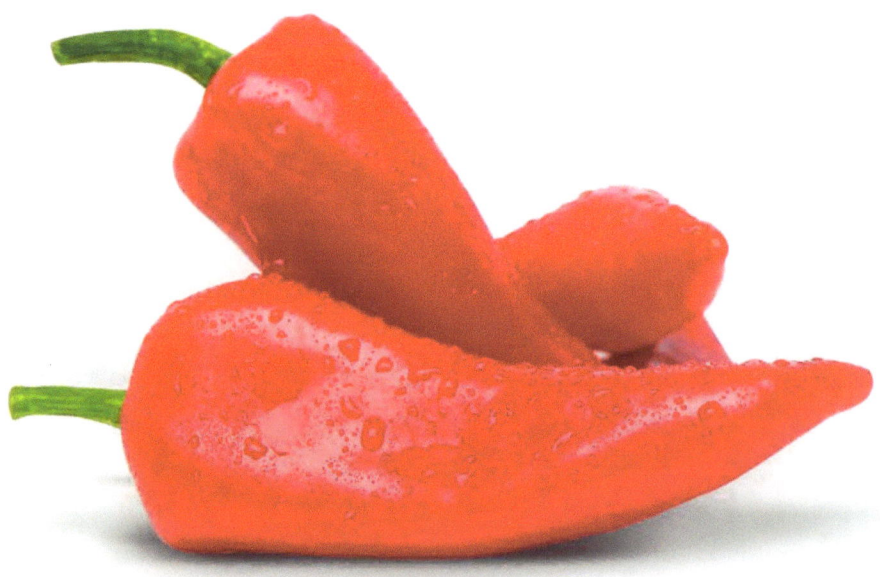

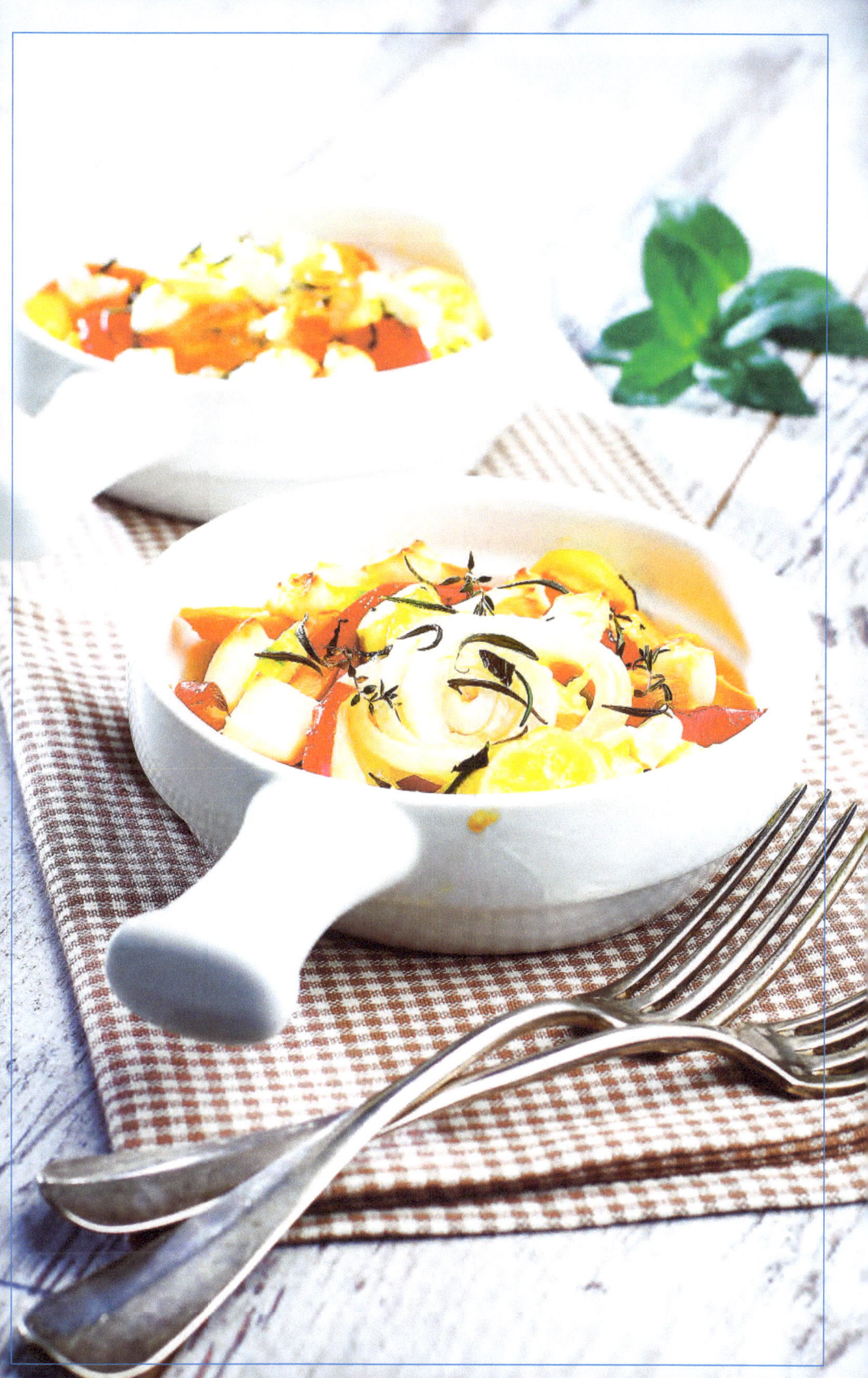

Pancakes

MAKES 6-7 SERVINGS

Ingredients

- 3 Eggs
- 115g Organic Whole Wheat Flour
- 1 Dessertspoon Baking Powder
- 140ml Milk
- A Pinch of Salt
- Coconut Oil

Directions

1. Make sure the eggs are at room temperature. Separate the yolks from the whites, place in a bowl and set aside.
2. Add a pinch of salt to the egg whites and beat well with a clean and dry mixer.
3. Within about 5 minutes, the egg whites will form foamy stiff peaks. Stop beating when the mixture is firm.
4. Into the bowl with the egg yolks, first add the milk, then the baking powder and the flour. Mix well.
5. Gently fold the beaten egg whites into the batter with a rubber spatula using a scooping and folding motion.
6. Set the batter aside and let sit for 5 minutes at room temperature.
7. Melt the coconut oil in a pan over medium heat.
8. Take a scoop of the batter and pour into the hot pan. Pancakes a half-centimeter thick are ideal.
9. Flip each pancake over with a spatula to cook the other side.

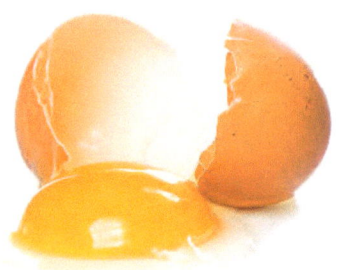

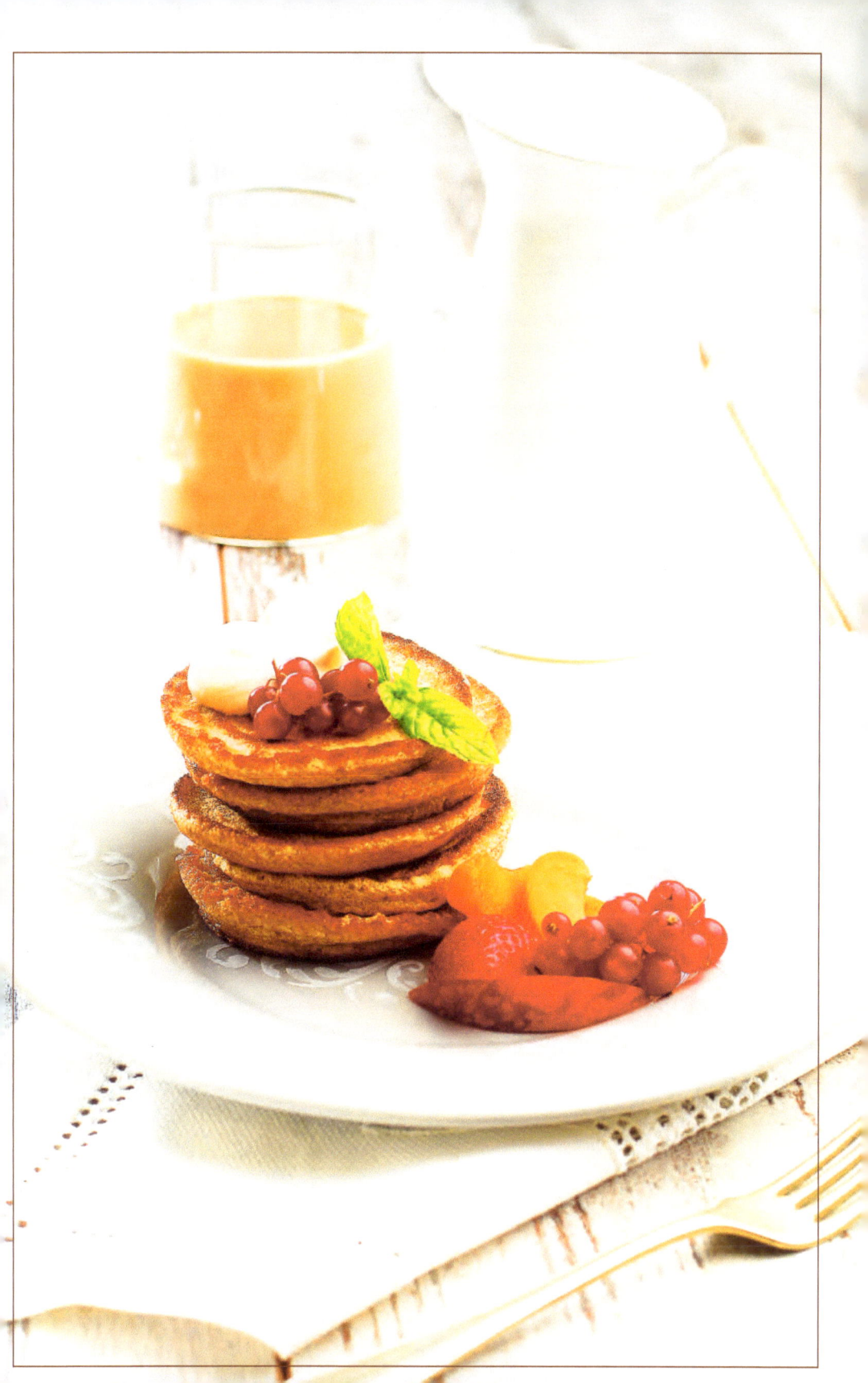

Veggie Pizza

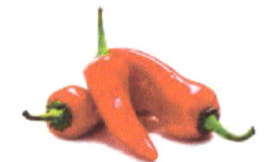

MAKES 1-2 SERVINGS

Ingredients

- 1 Whole Wheat Lavash
- 1 Zucchini
- 1 Small Sweet Red Pepper
- 4 Cherry Tomatoes
- 1 Large Garlic Clove
- Sea Salt
- Olive Oil
- 2 White Goat Cheddars, Grated

Directions

1. Spread a sheet of parchment paper on a baking tray and place the lavash on it.
2. Grate the garlic and mix with 1 tablespoon of olive oil. Smear this over the lavash.
3. Spread 1 tablespoon of grated cheddar cheese evenly over the lavash.
4. Peel and cut the zucchini into thin slices, and arrange over the cheese.
5. Cut the pizza into 8 equal slices.
6. Cut the red pepper into slices and cherry tomatoes into halves.
7. Place at least one slice of pepper and one tomato half on each slice.
8. Preheat the oven to 180C and bake the pizza until the veggies are soft.
9. Spread the rest of the cheese on top and bake for another 10 minutes.

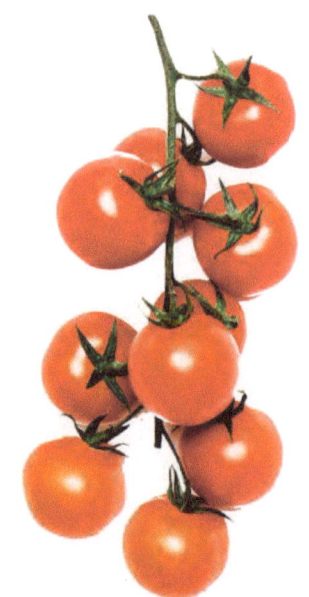

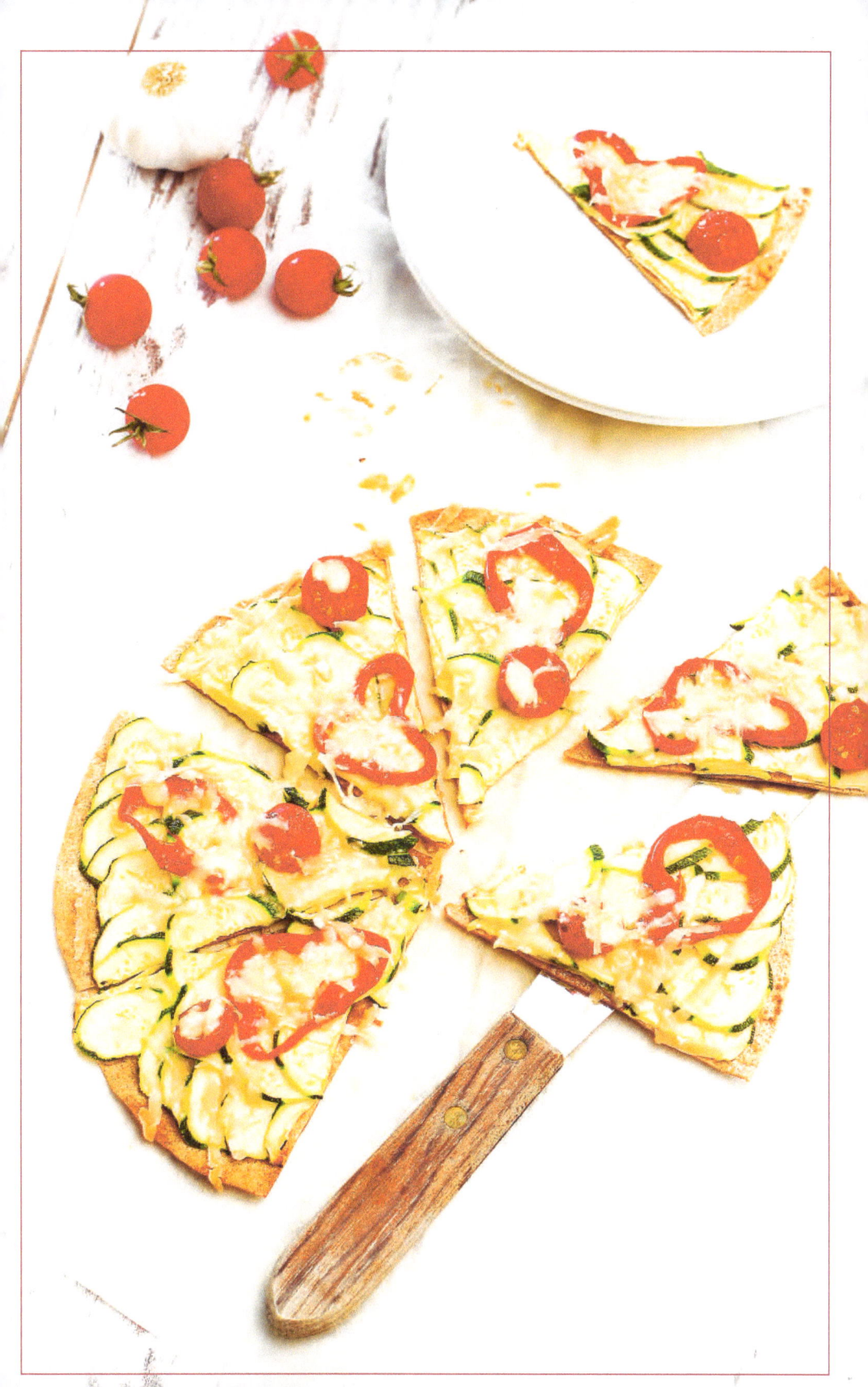

Sugar-Free Chocolate

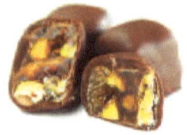

MAKES 4-5 SERVINGS

Ingredients

- 65ml Coconut Oil
- 130ml Cocoa
- 2 Dessertspoons Carob Flour
- 1 Dessertspoon Grape Molasses
- 1 Teaspoon Maca Powder
- 5-6 Cardamom Pods
- 1 Tablespoon Raisins
- 1 Tablespoon Raw Almonds

Directions

1. Mix all ingredients in a large bowl.
2. Spread a sheet of parchment paper on a baking tray and spread the mixture over the paper.
3. Place in the refrigerator and let sit for 2 hours.
4. Divide into small pieces.
5. Store in a lidded food storage container in the refrigerator until ready to be served.

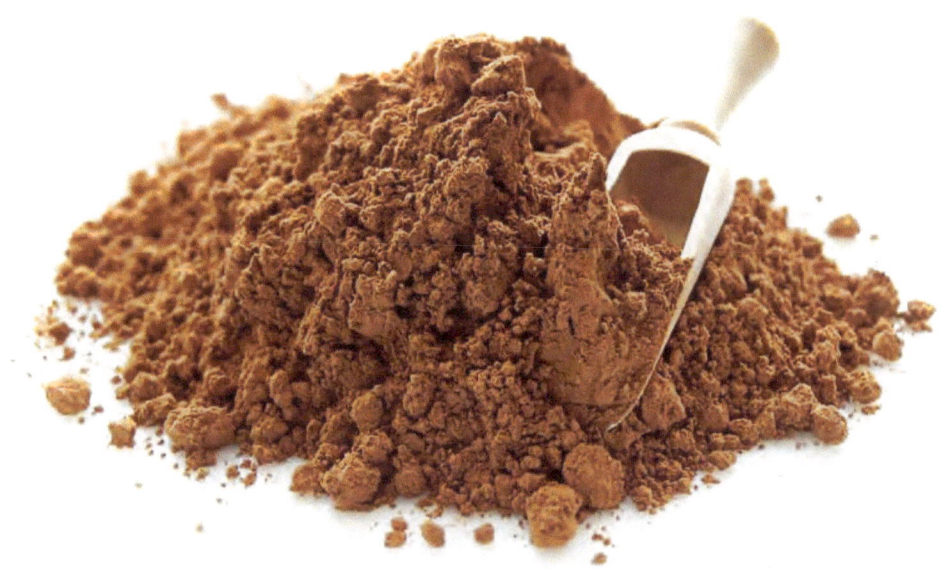

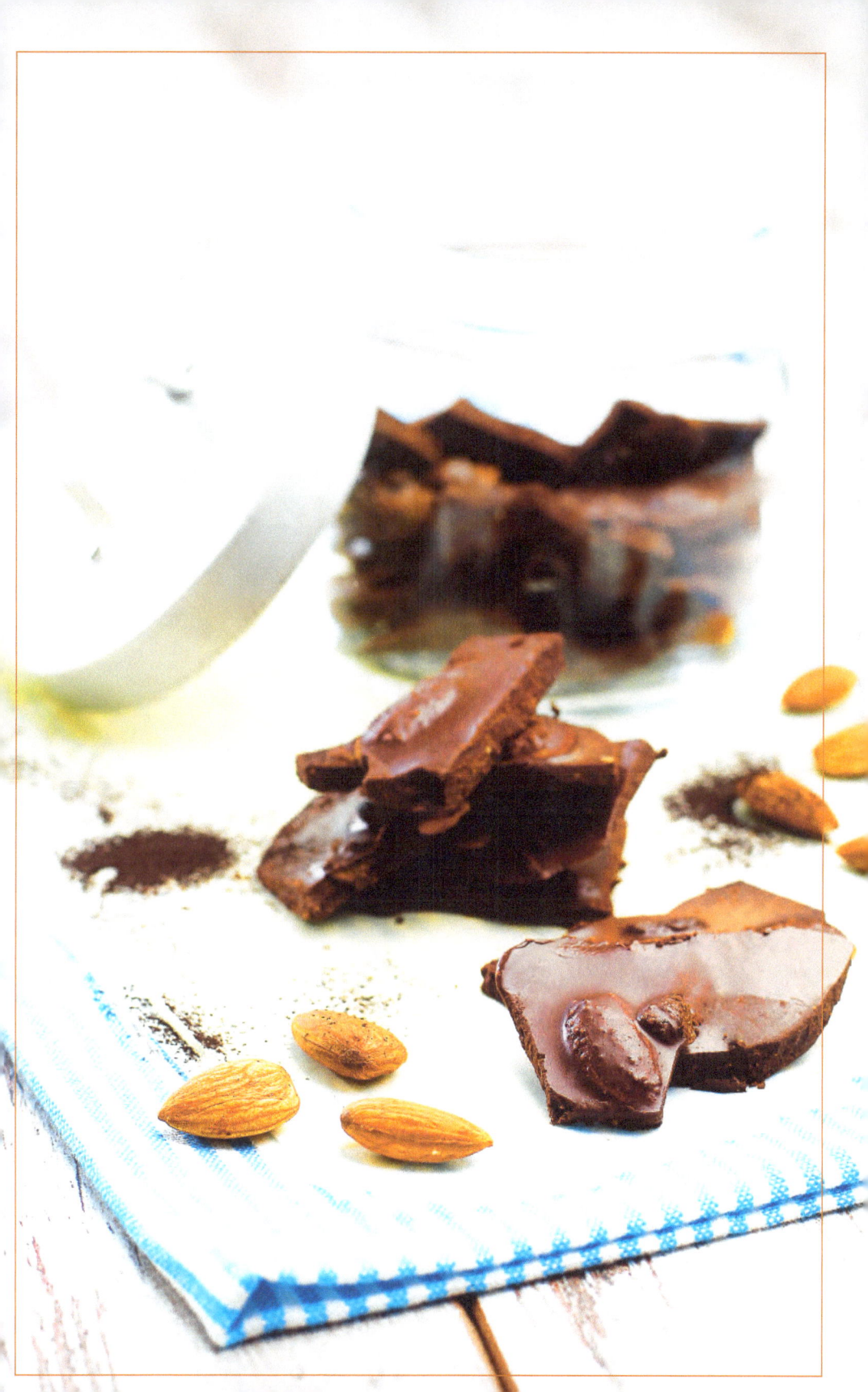

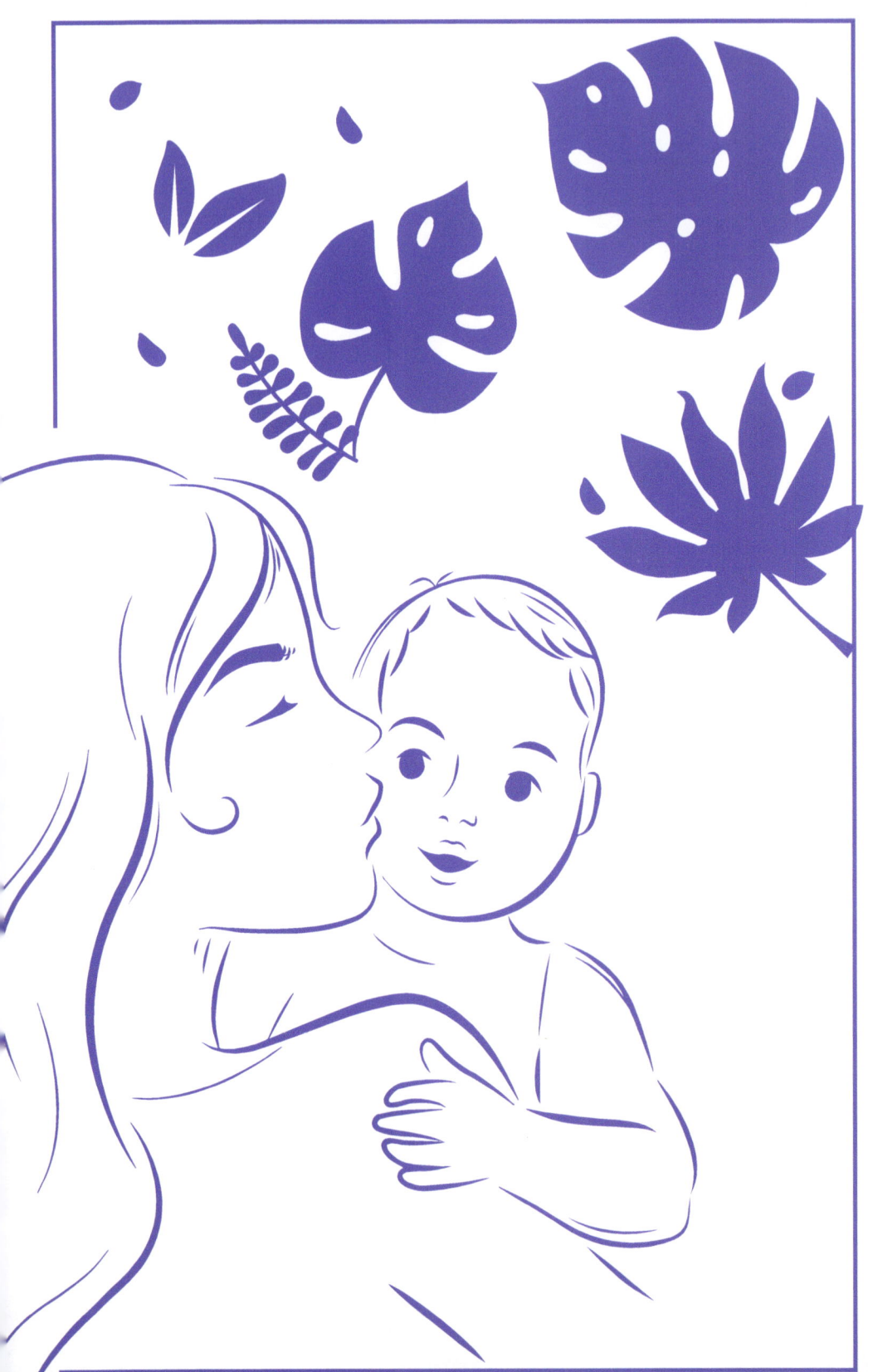

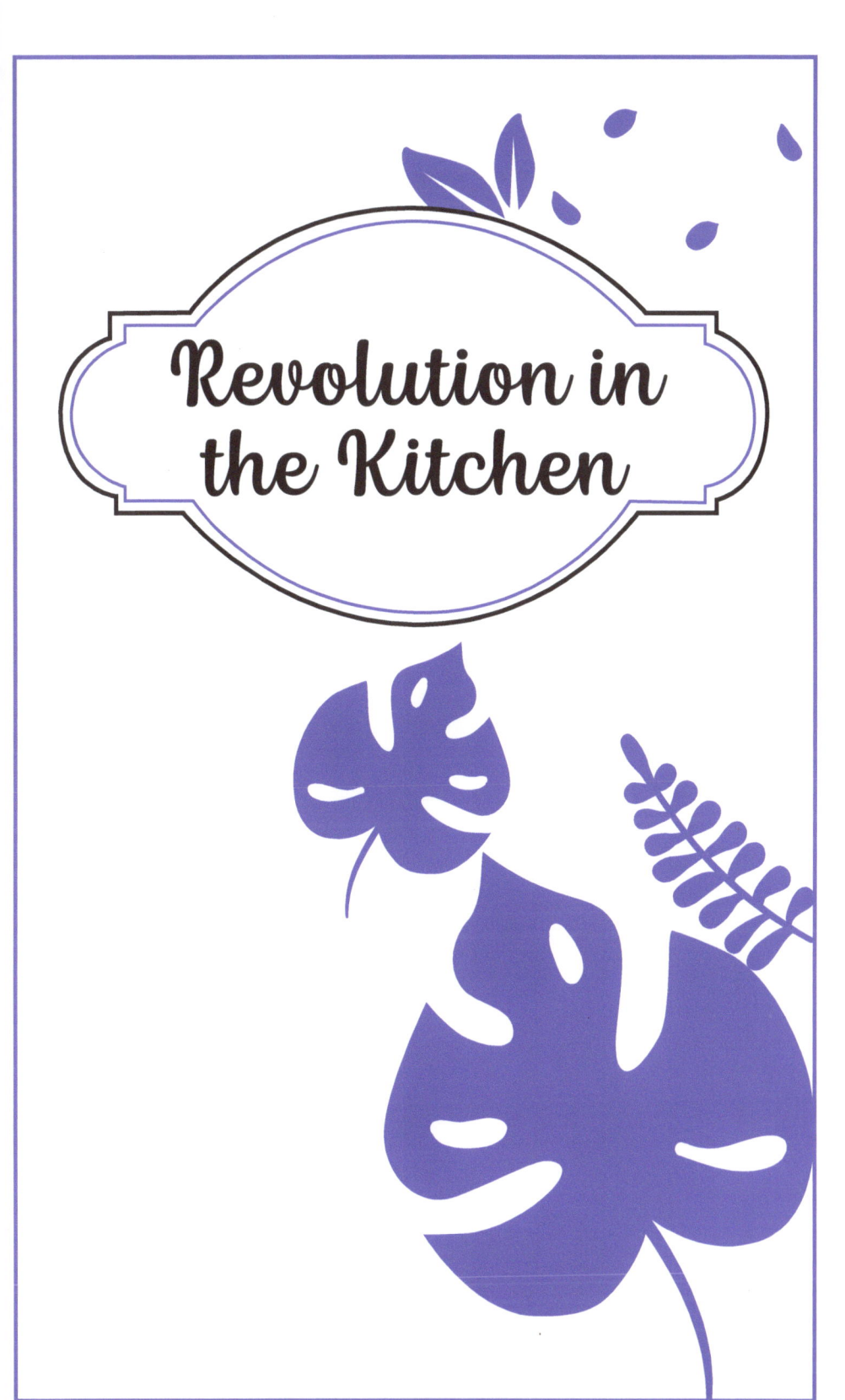

How to Make Bone Broth

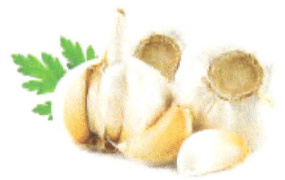

MAKES 6-8 SERVINGS

Ingredients

- Lamb Bones
- Drinking Water
- 1 Tablespoon Apple Cider Vinegar
- 1-2 Onions
- Garlic
- Whole Black Pepper
- 3-4 Bay Leaves

Directions

1. Place the lamb bones in a pot with water and other ingredients and boil for 5-6 hours.
2. Turn the heat off and allow the broth to cool.
3. Strain, discarding the bones. Pour into small storage containers and store in the freezer.

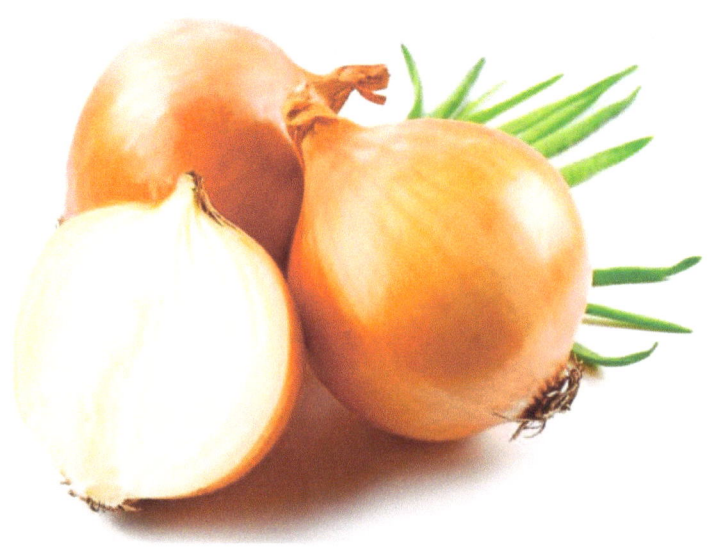

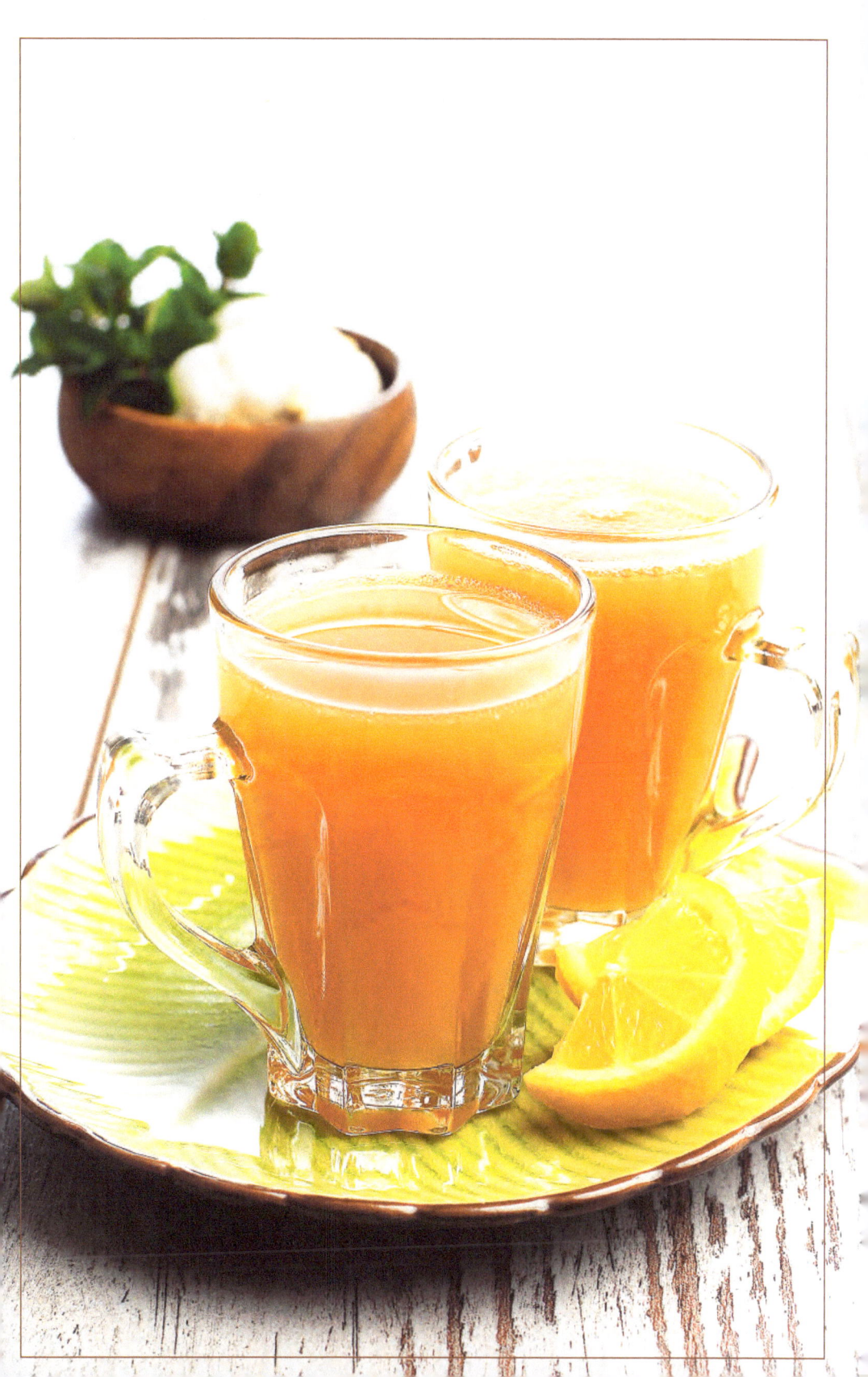

Ghee (Clarified Butter)

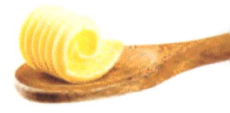

MAKES 6-8 SERVINGS

Ingredients

- 1kg Butter (or as much as you have)

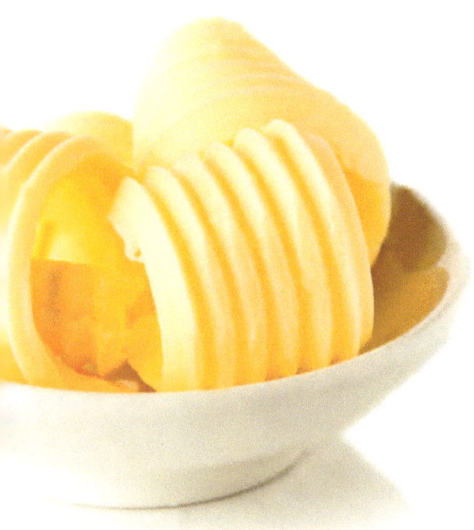

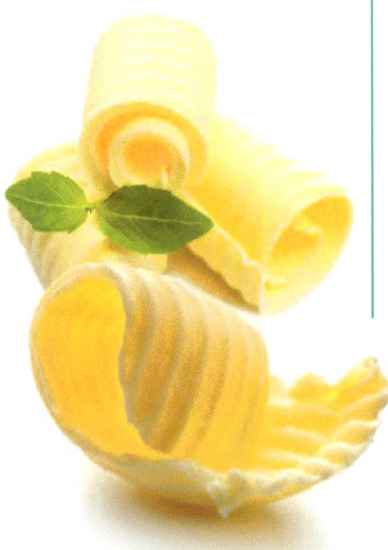

Directions

1. Place butter in a stainless-steel saucepan and melt over medium-low heat.
2. After melting, it will turn to a golden color.
4. Skim off the foam that appears on the top with a straining ladle.
5. Continue to cook the butter over low heat about 20-25 minutes. Make sure not to burn the butter.
6. Turn the heat off at the end of the cooking time.
7. Place clean cheesecloth in a large mesh strainer and carefully strain the ghee through cheesecloth into a mason jar.
8. After it cools to room temperature store in the refrigerator to keep it fresh for months.

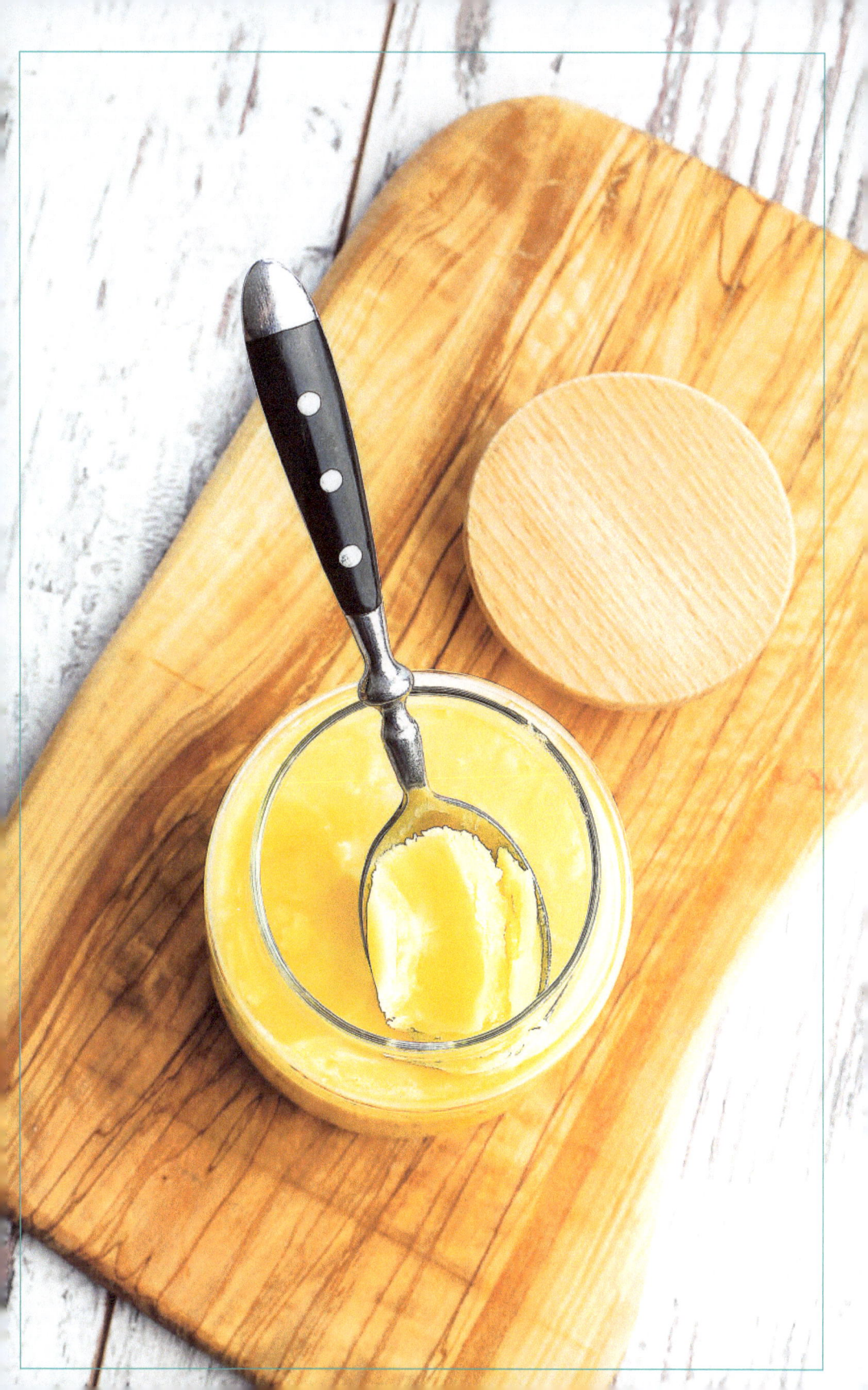

Homemade Yogurt

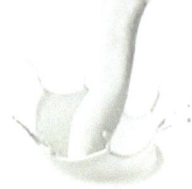

MAKES 6-8 SERVINGS

Ingredients

- 1 Liter Daily Milk
- 1 Tablespoon Yogurt (homemade preferred)
- Pinch of Salt

Directions

1. Boil the milk in a stainless steel pan over medium heat.
2. Continue the boiling process on low heat until almost a finger of the milk evaporates.
3. Turn the heat off and allow milk to cool for 10-15 minutes.
4. Dip your pinky finger in the milk to check the temperature.
5. If you can stand the heat, then it is cool enough to add the starter yogurt.
6. Place the starter yogurt in a small bowl, add salt and a little milk, stirring to make sure it's consistent.
7. Add the starter to the milk. Stir and mix thoroughly.
8. Pour this cultured milk into a glass jar or in a bowl with a lid. Wrap a kitchen towel tightly around the jar or the bowl to keep it warm.
9. Put it in a slightly warm area of the house where there's no air circulation and let it incubate. Your homemade yogurt should be ready in 3-4 hours.

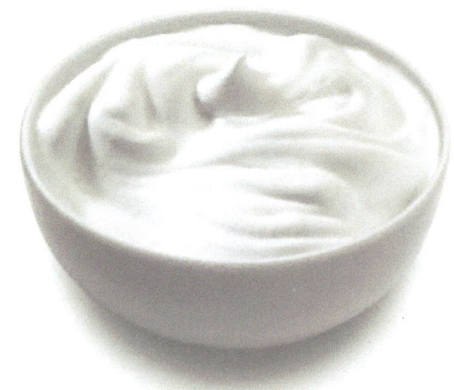

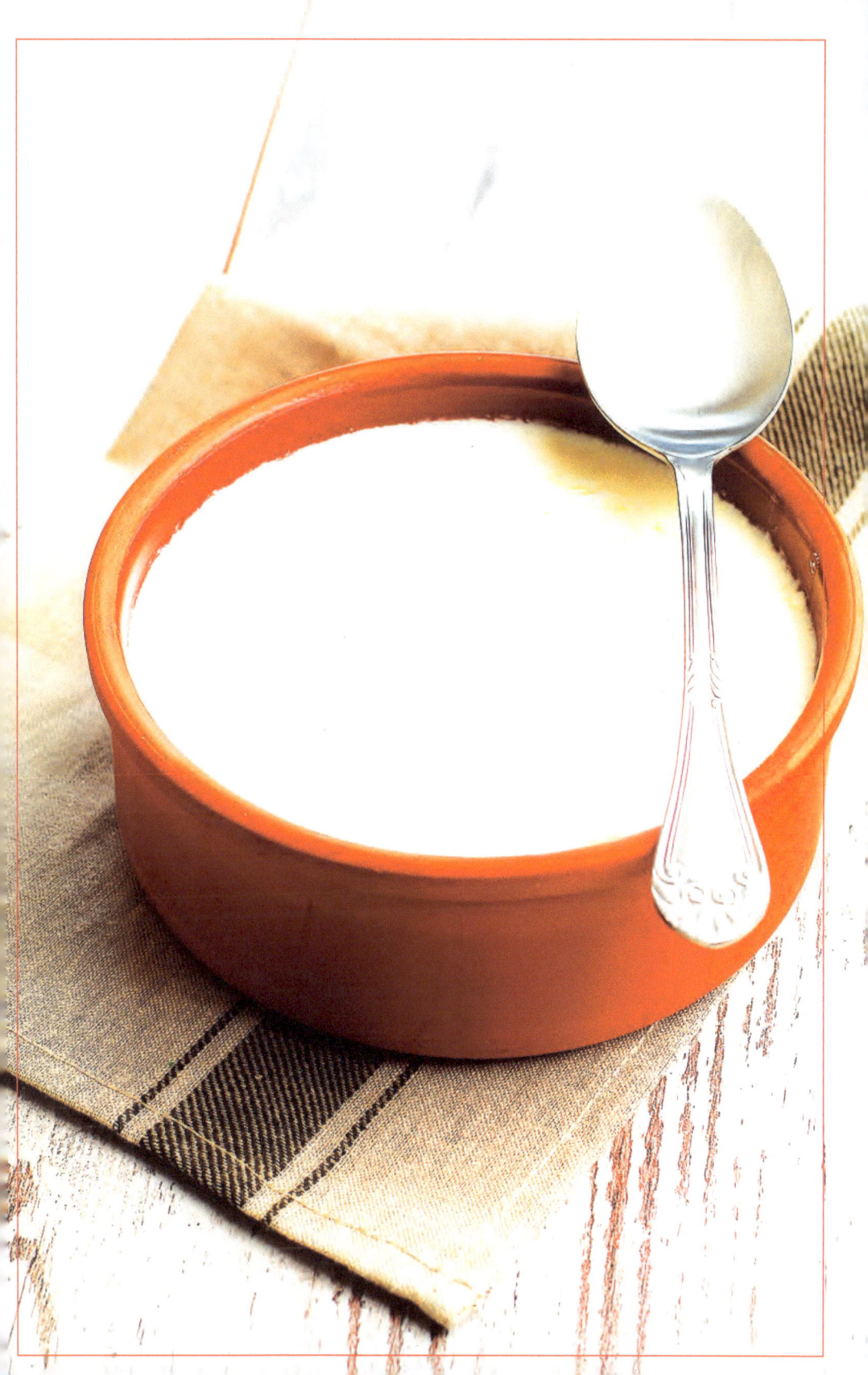

Coconut Milk

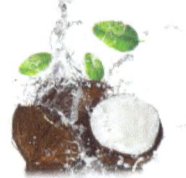

MAKES 6-8 SERVINGS

Ingredients

- 1 Coconut
- 600ml Hot Water

Directions

1. Crack open the coconut and scoop out the meat.
2. Add the coconut meat to a blender, pour 600ml hot water over it and blend for 5 minutes.
3. Allow it to cool.
4. Strain the liquid through a very fine cheesecloth.
5. Milk will keep in the refrigerator for 4-5 days.
6. You can use the coconut remains in the cheesecloth for desserts.

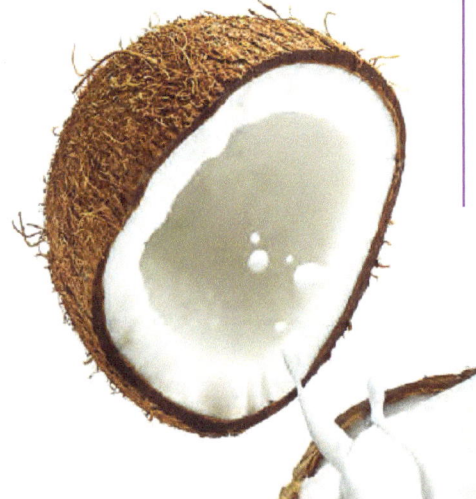

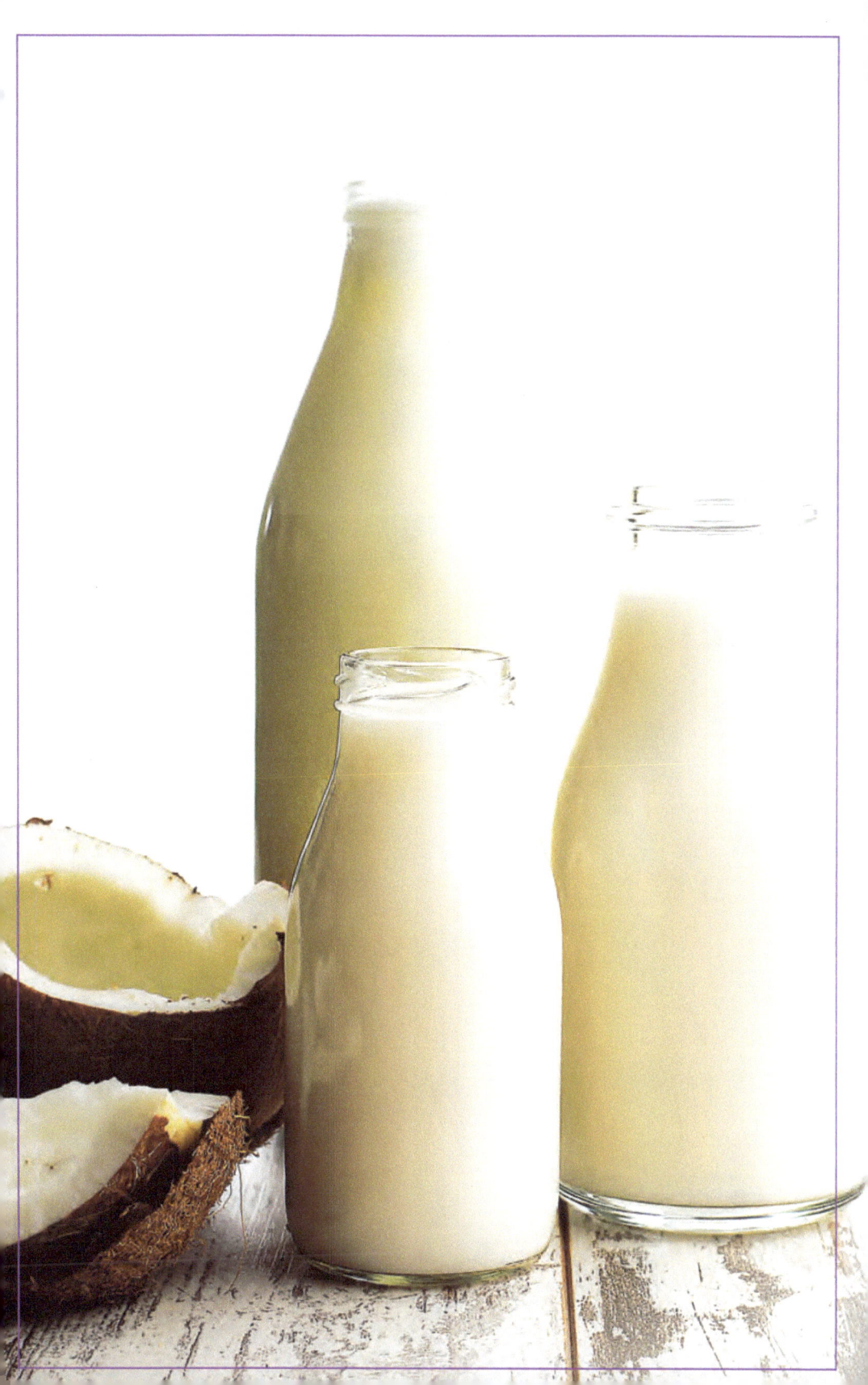

Almond Milk

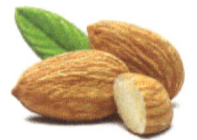

MAKES 6-8 SERVINGS

Ingredients

- 400ml Raw Almonds
- 1.2 Litres Water
- A Pinch Salt

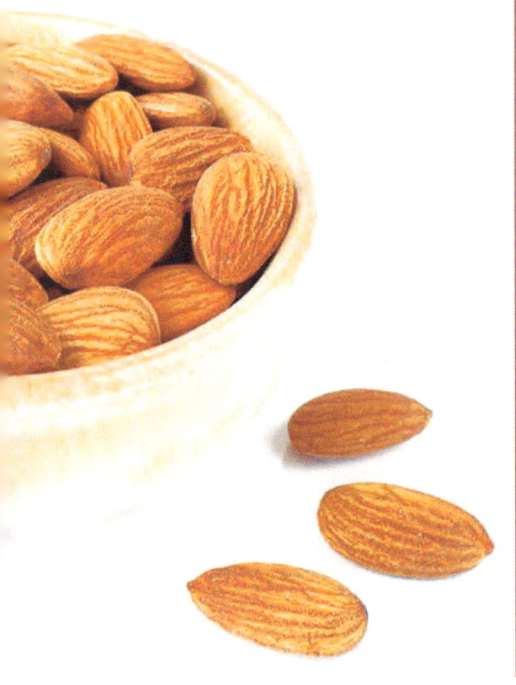

Directions

1. Put almonds in a glass jar and fill with enough water to cover.
2. Allow to sit at room temperature for 12 hours.
3. Drain the almonds when thetime is up.
4. In a blender, combine almonds with salt and 1.2 litres of water. Blend at high speed for 1-2 minutes.
5. Pour the mixture, including almonds, into a container and store in the refrigerator to avoid vitamin loss.
6. This will stay fresh in the refrigerator for 3 days.
7. If you want it to be like store-bought almond milk, you can strain the mixture before storing it.

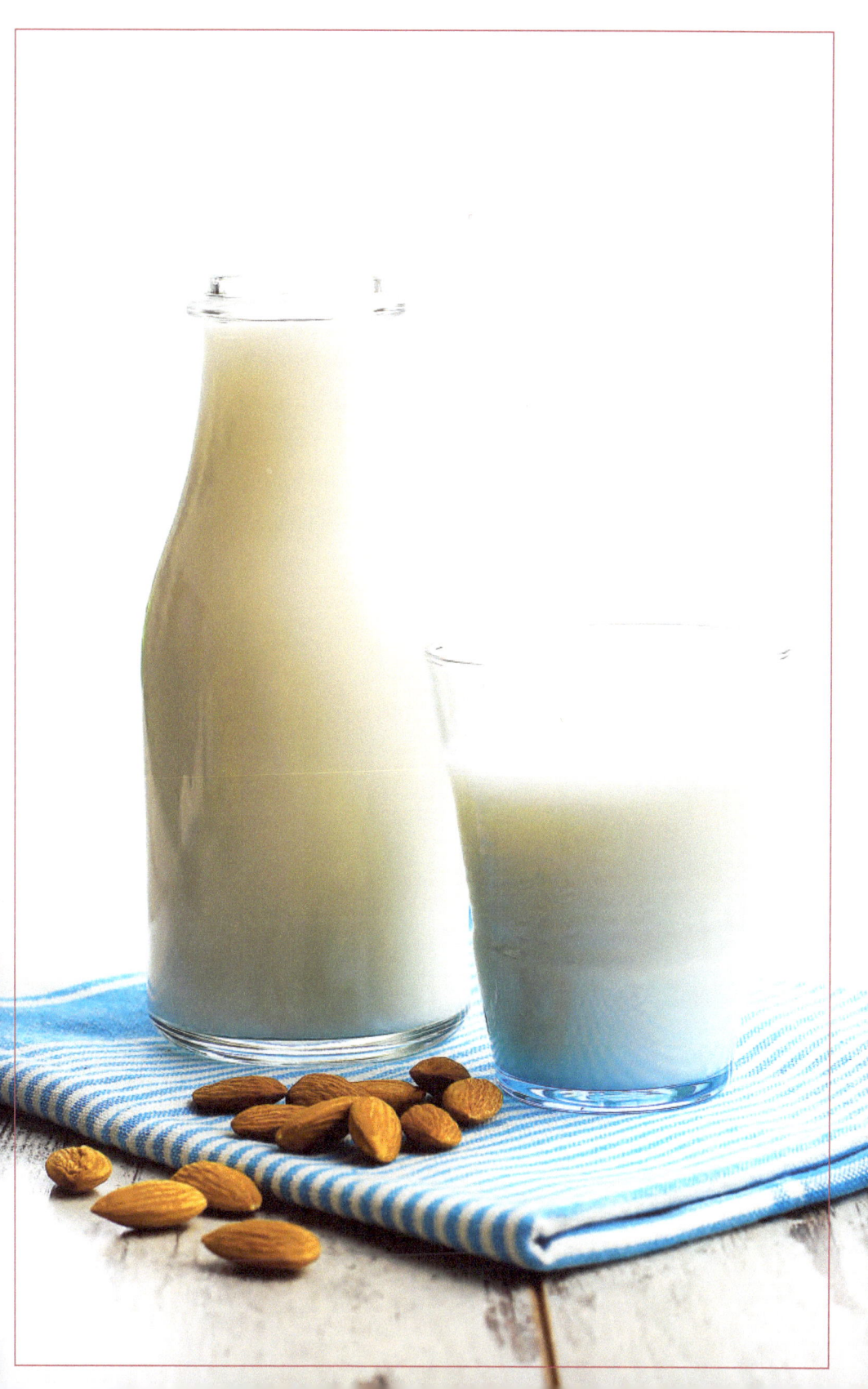

Easy Homemade Lemonade

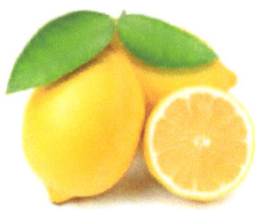

MAKES 6-8 SERVINGS

Ingredients

- 6-7 Organic Lemons
- 1 Liter Cold Water
- Honey, To Taste
- Mint Leaves

Directions

1. Wash the lemons well and juice lemons with their skin in a juicer.
2. Add honey and cold water, and mix well. Serve with fresh mint leaves.

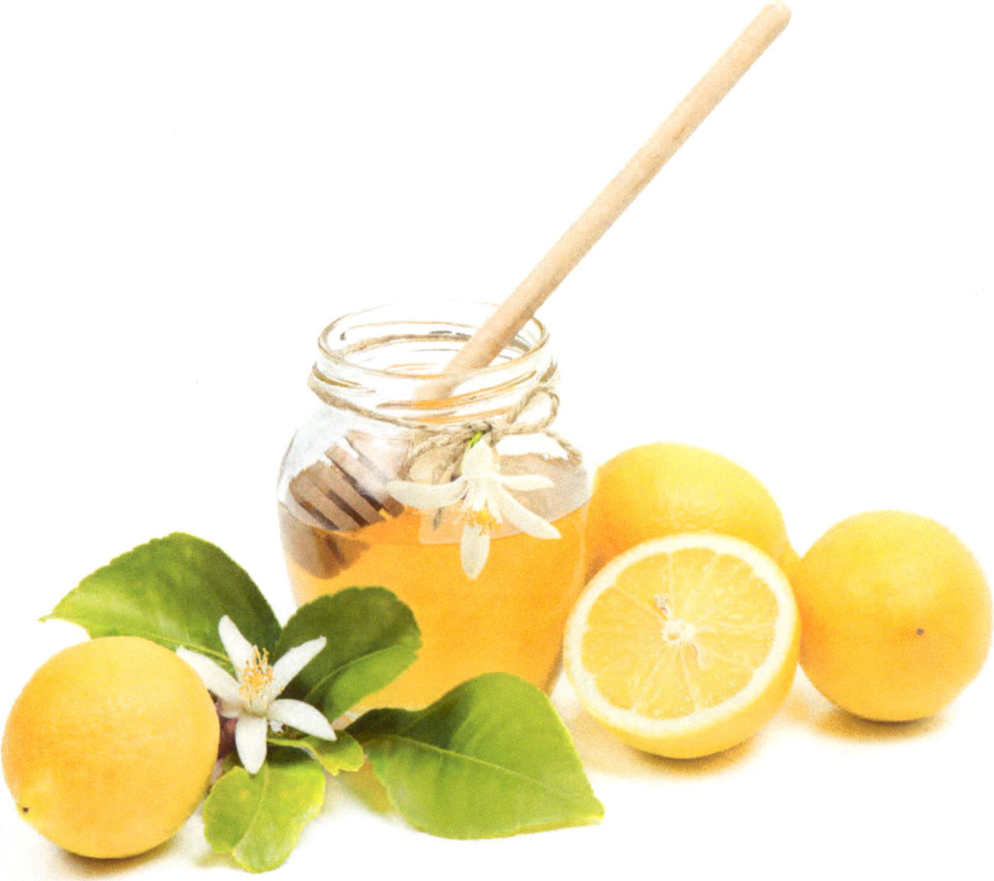

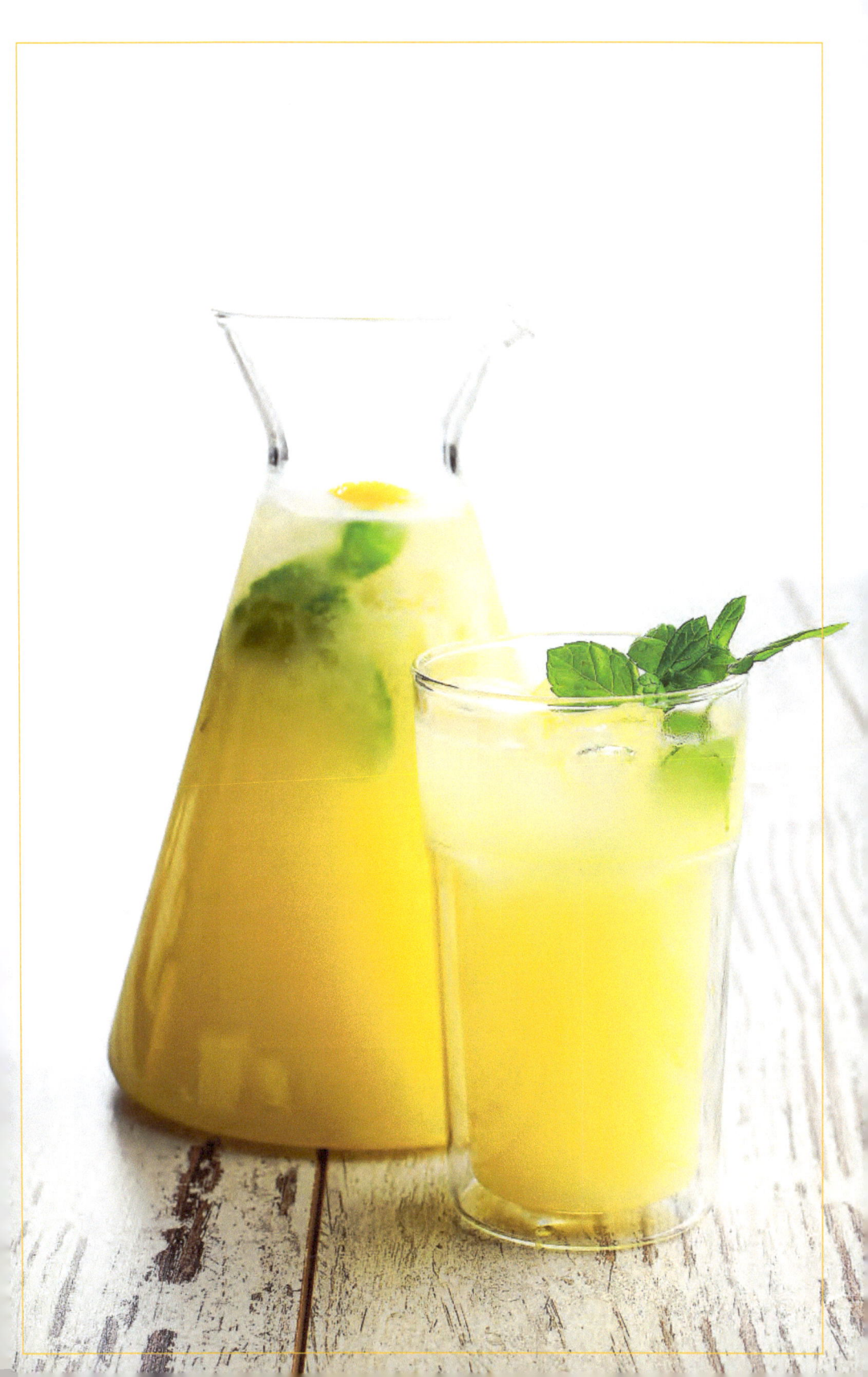

Homemade Ice Tea

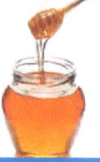

MAKES 6-8 SERVINGS

Ingredients

- 200ml Strong Tea
- 3 Lemons
- 1 Liter Water
- Mint Leaves
- Honey, To Your Taste

Directions

1. Squeeze the juice out of lemons, mix with tea and water.
2. Sweeten with honey and mint leaves to your taste.

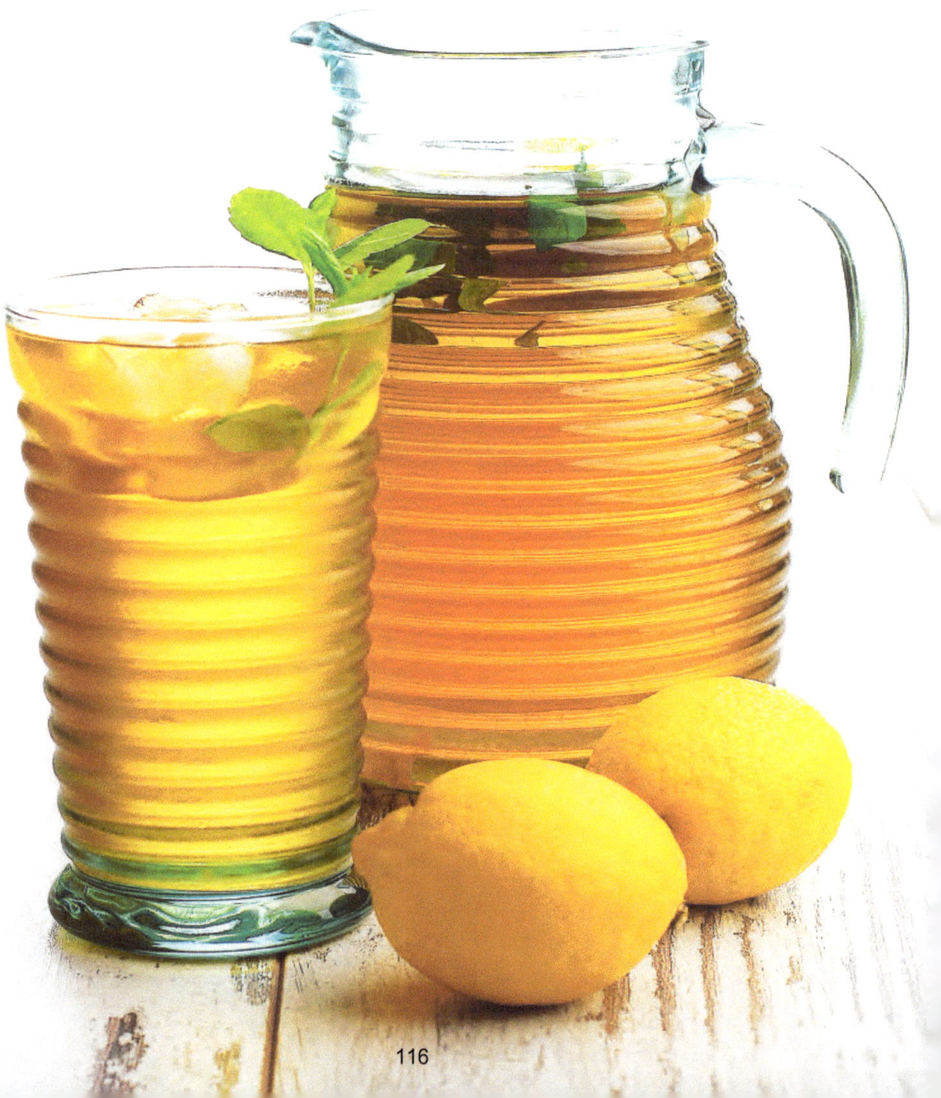

Habits to Change

OLD HABITS	NEW HABITS

www.ingramcontent.com/pod-product-compliance
Lightning Source LLC
Chambersburg PA
CBHW041621220426
43662CB00001B/8